VEINS

A Guide
to Prevention
and Treatment

FUNDS TO PURCHASE
THIS BOOK WERE
PROVIDED BY A
40TH ANNIVERSARY GRANT
FROM THE
FOELLINGER FOUNDATION.

VARICOSE VEINS

A Guide
to Prevention
and Treatment

Howard C. Baron, M.D., F.A.C.S.

and

Barbara A. Ross

Facts On File, Inc.

Varicose Veins: A Guide to Prevention and Treatment

Facts On File, Inc.
11 Penn Plaza
New York, NY 10001

Library of Congress Cataloging-in-Publication Data
Baron, Howard C.
Varicose veins: a guide to prevention and treatment / Howard C. Baron and Barbara A. Ross.
p. cm.
Includes index.
ISBN 0-8160-3652-7 (acid-free paper)
1. Varicose veins. I. Ross, Barbara A. II. Title.
RC695.B343 1995
616.1'43—dc20

Facts On File books are available at special discounts when purchased in bulk quantities for businesses, associations, institutions or sales promotions. Please call our Special Sales Department in New York at 212/967-8800 or 800/322-8755

Cover design by Dorothy Wachtenheim

This book is printed on acid-free paper.

Printed in the United States of America

VB FOF   First paperback printing February 1997

CONTENTS

INTRODUCTION

It has been 15 years since I last wrote a book for the lay public on varicose veins. The purpose of this book remains largely unchanged: to give readers the information they need to know about diseases of the vascular system in a concise, readable form. I also want to bring readers up-to-date about the diagnosis and treatment of varicose and spider veins and the causes of them.

The subject is becoming increasingly relevant as the American population ages. By the end of this decade, 21 million baby boomers will be reaching their 50s, the age when varicose veins start showing up in large numbers, particularly in women. It is estimated that at least 25% of all American women have varicose veins, and the number grows as the women age. By the time they reach their 60s, an estimated 72% of American women will experience varicose veins. Men are not immune from them, either. An estimated 42% of all American men over 60 get varicose veins. And according to the most definitive study ever done on the subject, the number of people developing varicose veins in Western civilization is growing.

Most consider the unsightly blue bulges and spider marks on the legs to be a mere cosmetic nuisance, but each year approximately 150,000 Americans die of related complications and 2.5 million others are severely disabled by them.

In the chapters that follow, the basics of what you need to know about the circulatory system, the symptoms of varicose veins (that are often ignored by people with busy lifestyles), the suspected and proven causes of varicose veins and the treatments for them are given.

I also have expanded and updated the discussion of the reasons varicose veins seem to affect women more than men, by a factor of four to one or more. Chapter 7 also gives you the latest research on the impact of oral contraceptives and hormone replacement therapies on your veins. Finally, I offer some commonsense advice for avoiding varicose veins.

Although varicose veins are far more common in Western industrialized countries, they are not new. One of the earliest papyri from ancient Egypt, a medical text written 3,000 years before the birth of Christ, discusses the problem. Ancient Greek physicians were also aware of it. A votive relief of a leg showing varicose veins can be seen in the National Museum of Athens.

Scientists and practitioners who specialize in this field have learned a lot about the problem. In the last 15 years, for example, researchers believe they have isolated a gene that causes varicose veins in some people. Meanwhile, vascular surgeons, using and improving on advances in medical technology, are making smaller incisions and removing smaller segments of leg veins than they used to and much of the surgery is being done without expensive overnight hospital stays. By removing shorter vein segments, we have been able to leave veins in the legs and harvest them later, if necessary, for use in by-pass surgery. There also have been advances in the diagnosis of varicose veins with devices that use sonar and other technologies. In addition, vascular surgeons, including this author, are developing new techniques for repairing malfunctioning vein valves. If these pioneering techniques prove successful, doctors will be able to remove even shorter vein segments to cure varicose veins. It is time for the lay public to be informed of these advances and to know more, in general, about vascular diseases that strike millions of people but do not generate as much media attention as arterial diseases.

There are several reasons why you need to know more about vascular diseases.

One, the symptoms of varicose veins are often missed or misinterpreted by general practitioners.

Two, when varicose and spider veins are visible, patients are unsure if they should go to a dermatologist or a surgeon. Normally (and preferably), patients are referred to one or the other by their family doctor, but all too often they go directly to a specialist. This book will help you decide which is appropriate for your needs.

Finally, in this age of managed health care where insurance companies are disallowing many legitimate claims in order to keep expenses down, it has become increasingly important for people to learn more about their health. Patients who are knowledgeable will not easily be denied their rights to decent health care by someone with minimal or no medical training to determine what, if any, treatment is necessary.

For example, I'll bet many feminist leaders (and male lawmakers who court women's votes) don't know that Medicare will reimburse older people for vascular treatment only if they are diagnosed as having varicose veins with inflammation, varicose veins with ulcers or varicose veins with both ulcers and inflammation. When you read Chapter 6 on potentially serious complications that come with varicose veins, you will understand that Medicare's policy effectively means they will allow treatment only *after* a patient's condition has deteriorated.

Medicare also has repeatedly cut the percentage that it will reimburse doctors and hospitals for treatment of vascular problems. That means that a lot of elderly women who can't afford supplemental health insurance have to spend much of their limited income to maintain their health. Since it is a fact that varicose veins strike far more women than men, these Medicare policies might make a fine cause for *knowledgeable* women to fight.

The same kind of discrimination is occurring with younger women in the workforce who have private health insurance. I recently had two patients in their late 20s, one man, one woman. They had the same problem requiring the same operation, and although they had different employers, they were covered by the same insurance company. However, the man had a more expensive, more complete insurance policy. The insurance company determined that he needed the surgery and she did not and it refused to pay for her operation.

Vascular specialists also are seeing this problem increasingly crop up with patients covered by health maintenance organizations. HMOs almost always refuse to pay for any kind of sclerotherapy (a process that involves multiple chemical injections in varicose veins), arguing that it is being done for cosmetic, not medical, reasons. In fact, it's often performed in combination with surgery for very serious medical reasons and it also is done as an office procedure without surgery for valid reasons. These policies are creating a public health problem because patients are being forced to forego treatment until serious complications set in. It is estimated that two million hours of work per year are lost in this country each year because of varicose ulcers. If the varicose veins causing these ulcers had been treated properly in a timely way, there would have been no need for this loss in productivity—not to mention the suffering of those in pain.

This book offers the information you need to determine whether you have a vascular condition serious enough to warrant medical attention, to understand the recommended medical procedures and to know what reimbursement you are entitled to from your insurance carrier.

My co-author and I would like to thank our friends and associates for their advice and generous assistance, particularly Dr. John Bergan, Dr. J. Leonel Villavicencio, Dr. Mitchel Goldman, Dr. Lila Nachtigall, Suzanne Gluck of ICM, our Medical illustrator Shirley Baty, and our spouses.

—Howard C. Baron, M.D., F.A.C.S.
Associate Professor of Surgery,
N.Y.U. School of Medicine
Attending Vascular Surgeon,
Cabrini Medical Center
New York, New York

VARICOSE VEINS

A Guide to Prevention and Treatment

CHAPTER 1

■ ■

THE CIRCULATORY
SYSTEM

Almost one in seven Americans has a disease involving some part of the circulatory system. A failure of that system accounts for 53% of all deaths in America. Varicose veins is just one kind of vascular disease, but it is the most common.

One in four women in the United States has varicose veins. Ten times more people suffer from diseases of the veins than from diseases of the arteries. Last year, more than 150,000 Americans died from a complication of venous diseases; another 2.5 million were severely disabled.

To understand varicose veins, it is essential to know something about the way that blood (approximately six quarts) constantly moves through your circulatory system and about each of that system's major players—your heart, arteries and veins.

The start of the circulatory system is the heart, which beats about 70 times a minute, pumps about 4,000 gallons of blood a day and beats 2.5 billion times in an average lifetime. When something happens to the heart, the effect can be very dramatic. It often means sudden death. A shock can stop it. A clot can cut off its blood supply. Coronary arteries, which bring oxygenated blood to the heart muscles, can narrow and strangle it.

Arteries carry blood away from the heart. When something happens to arteries, the effects can also be devastating. Blood flows through the arteries under enormous pressure. When an artery is punctured, the blood spurts out, and usually requires emergency medical attention.

In contrast, veins, which return blood to the heart, seem to do nothing dramatic; they just work. It is hard to become excited about them until you realize they cause more problems for more people

1

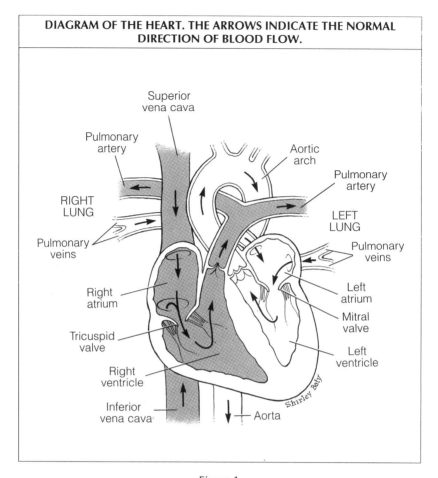

DIAGRAM OF THE HEART. THE ARROWS INDICATE THE NORMAL DIRECTION OF BLOOD FLOW.

Figure 1

than all the heart and artery problems combined—annoying problems that can strike at any time.

The circulatory system works like this:

At the center of the system is the heart, a hollow muscle the size of a clenched fist. Its shape is like an ice cream cone; its broad top is tilted back and to the right and its downward point is directed forward and to the left.

The heart's job is to nourish and supply every part of the body with blood. In a person at rest, it pumps almost six quarts of blood per minute, but it can increase that amount by six to eight times for those engaged in strenuous exercise.

SCHEMATIC DIAGRAM OF THE CIRCULATORY SYSTEM OF THE BODY.

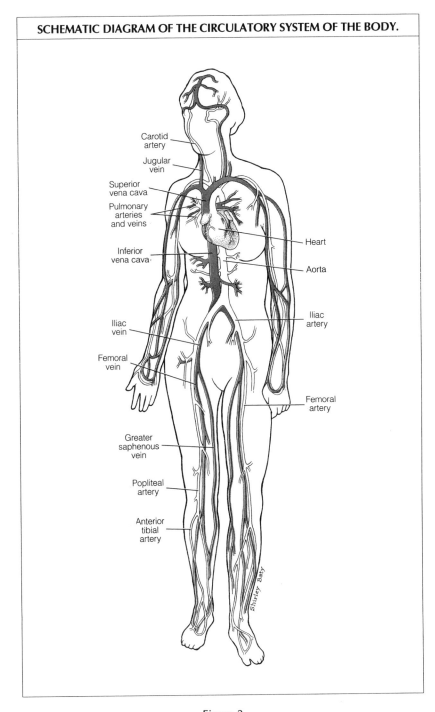

Figure 2

The heart has four chambers: two that accept blood (auricles) and two that eject blood (ventricles). The auricles are on the top of the heart, the ventricles on the bottom.

The chambers are separated by valves that allow blood to flow in only one direction. When the valves do not operate properly and blood seeps the wrong way, it can be heard in a stethoscope as a heart murmur, a potentially dangerous condition.

Veins return blood from the body to the right upper heart, the right auricle. The blood then flows down into the right lower heart, the right ventricle, where it is pumped to the lungs. The lungs add oxygen, remove carbon dioxide and send the blood back to the left upper heart, or left auricle. It flows down to the left lower heart, or left ventricle, where it is pumped into the aorta, the largest artery in the body. No one is quite sure why the heart works, but it is remarkable.

The aorta is the main artery leading from the heart to the body. It is about one inch wide and has a thick wall of muscle fibers, one layer running lengthwise and one circular layer, allowing it to expand and contract in both length and diameter. Like other arteries, the aorta expands and contracts with each pulsation from a heart contraction.

From the aorta, the arteries branch into ever smaller units. Eventually, they connect with capillaries.

Capillaries are so tiny that they can be seen only with a microscope. They are so narrow, having a diameter that is one-tenth the thickness of a straight pin, that red cells move through them in single file. However, capillaries are so numerous in your body that if they were laid end to end, they would stretch around the world twice and still have enough length to make two round trips between New York and Los Angeles.

The capillaries act as brakes on the strong pressure from the arteries. Blood flows into the capillaries like a torrent; it leaves them like a gentle stream when it flows into the veins. Capillaries have an important job: They connect the arterioles (the smallest arteries) with the venules (the tiniest veins).

The cells that make up capillary walls also perform an important task: They take oxygen and nutrients from the blood and return carbon dioxide and other waste products of metabolism. Once the blood leaves the capillary system, it is venous blood. And now the process is reversed, so the blood can be oxygenated for use. From tiny veins, the blood flows into larger and larger ones until it all joins in the two main veins to the heart, the superior and inferior vena cavas.

THE ANATOMY OF THE GREATER SAPHENOUS VEIN AND ITS MOST CONSTANT TRIBUTARIES.

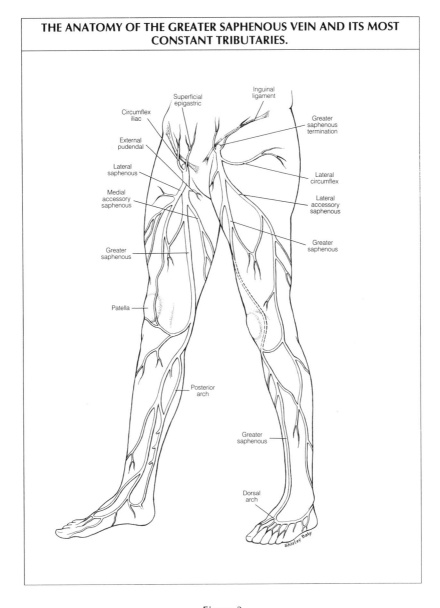

Figure 3

THE ANATOMY OF THE LESSER SAPHENOUS VEIN.

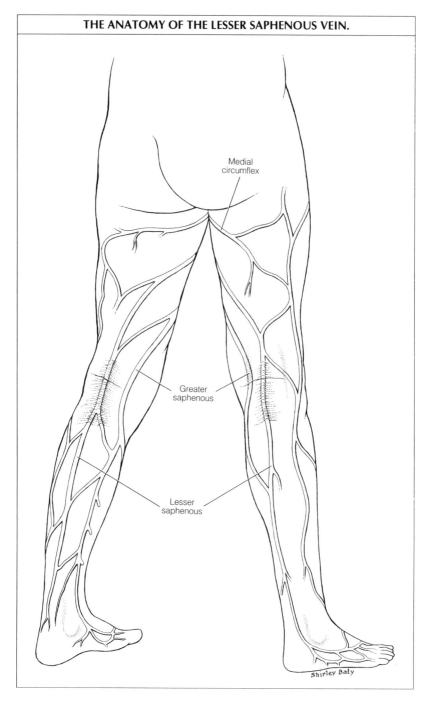

Figure 4

Arteries and veins have an equally important role in the circulatory system; they also are similarly constructed. For example, both have inner, middle and external layers. However, arteries are fed by the heart while veins are fed by clusters of capillaries. Also, veins might be considered more vulnerable because they have thinner walls; their middle coat is less well developed and less elastic; and many veins have valves which can malfunction.

One final note: If connected end to end, the various arteries, arterioles, capillaries, venules and veins in your body would stretch some 70,000 miles. Yet, despite the distance it travels, and the circuitous route it follows, the blood leaving your heart at this instant should be back in your heart in 23 seconds.

Varicose and spider veins almost always occur in the legs. The two leg veins you have to know the most about are called the greater and lesser saphenous veins. The greater saphenous vein is the longest vein in the body, running from the inside of the ankle up to the groin. There it meets the femoral vein which runs into the iliac vein in the pelvis. The iliac then joins the vena cava which travels to the heart.

The lesser saphenous vein begins on the outside of the ankle and curves up behind the knee. Here it joins with the popliteal vein and continues back to the heart.

Both saphenous veins are located in the layer of fat just beneath the skin.

The other two important leg veins are the deep veins and perforator veins. Deep veins run alongside the arteries and are protected by fibrous tissue and muscles. Perforator veins that connect the saphenous and deep veins also are surrounded by muscles and dense fibrous tissue. The number of perforator veins varies from person to person. Some have two, others as many as six. Most of the important perforator veins are located in the lower leg between the knee and ankle.

That's the basic roadmap.

The driving force that moves blood through your arteries is the pressure created by your pumping heart. When a doctor tells you that your blood pressure is 120 over 80, it means your arteries are under 120 millimeters of mercury pressure when your heart is contracting and 80 millimeters when your heart is at rest. The first is the systolic phase, the second the diastolic. When your systolic

DIAGRAM OF THE IMPORTANT COMMUNICATING (PERFORATOR) VEINS OF THE LEG THAT CONNECT THE SUPERFICIAL VEINS WITH THE DEEP VEINS.

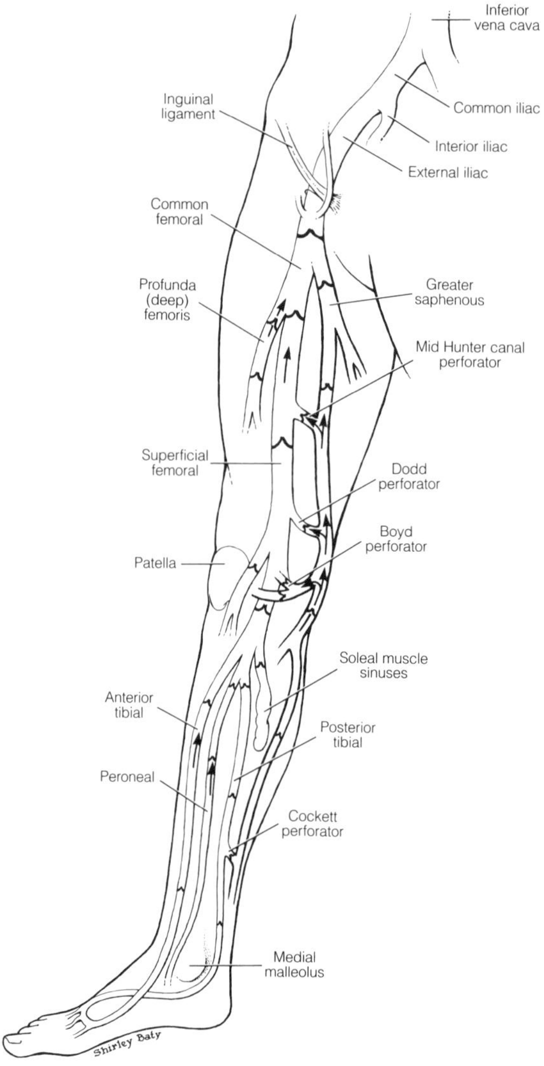

Figure 5

pressure is 120, it means your heart is contracting and pumping out blood with enough pressure to force a column of mercury in a tube to rise approximately 120 millimeters high.

Each heart contraction in a person with normal blood pressure can generate enough force to raise a column of mercury five to six inches high in a glass tube or five feet in a column of water. (Doctors measure blood pressure with a sphygmomanometer, a mercury-filled device because mercury is 13 ½ times heavier than water. If they used a water-filled device, they would need a 12-foot tube of water to measure a patient with high blood pressure.) This extraordinary pressure explains how blood travels through the arteries. With each contraction, it is being pushed by the muscular force of the left ventricle.

Blood pressure in the veins is generally much lower than it is in the arteries. For example, blood pressure in the branchial artery of your arm would normally be about 120/80 mm of mercury pressure but a vein in the same arm could be only 8 mm when the person is lying down. So, what makes blood come back through the veins?

Several factors are at work here.

First, there is the vacuum force created by the movement of your chest wall and diaphragm. The continuous movement of air every time you inhale and exhale creates a negative pressure or partial vacuum that helps blood return to the heart. The sucking action of the chest is mainly the result of the diaphragm, a powerful muscle that expands and contracts with your breathing, 20 to 30 times per minute, night and day.

A second factor involves the valves in your veins. They are found in your saphenous, deep and perforator veins. The valves—particularly in leg veins—make sure that your blood moves only toward the heart and upward against the flow of gravity. The valves also help spread the workload in veins throughout the lower extremities, particularly by preventing an abnormal rise in pressure in the saphenous veins.

The third force helping blood to return to your heart involves the muscles that surround your deep veins. As the muscles contract with exercise or regular movement, they squeeze the veins and force blood upward and back to the heart.

Varicose veins result when the vein valves stop working properly and blood in the venous system starts flowing in the wrong direction—away from the heart.

It therefore makes sense to look more closely at how those valves work. Valves are minute cuplike structures attached to both sides of inner vein walls. They begin to appear in the venules that carry blood away from the capillary beds. Although some veins do not have any valves and some have valves that are rudimentary and nonfunctional, leg veins are richly supplied with valves. They are located at strategically placed intervals in saphenous, deep and perforator veins.

Valves are most numerous in saphenous veins, but their numbers and location vary from person to person. Some have as few as six valves in the greater saphenous, others as many as 25. Similarly, the number in the lesser saphenous veins can run from 4 to 13. Generally, the more valves you have, the less chance you will develop a damaging backflow of blood that can cause a varicose vein. One study has shown, for example, that people with a normal great saphenous vein have valves every 3.5 inches compared to one every 6.5 inches for those with varicosities. Everybody has at least one valve in the five to six perforator veins between the knee and ankle.

Think of each vein valve as a pair of heavy curved church doors. When blood flows through a healthy vein at normal pressure, those doors are wide open or slightly ajar at the center, forming an arrowhead that points toward the heart. But at the first sign of increased venous pressure or wrong-way blood flow, the valves snap shut and no reasonable amount of pressure from behind the doors, or above the valves, can open them. In fact, the more pressure applied from the wrong side, the tighter the valves are closed.

Vein valves do more than direct the flow of blood back to the heart. Their most important function is to prevent a backflow of blood which could seriously damage your veins. Valves do this by dividing your leg veins into many individual, watertight chambers. There are more chambers (and valves) near your feet and fewer in the upper part of the thigh. These chambers are important because they allow veins, particularly in the lower extremities, to do their work gradually, relaxing between each push against gravity.

When valves fail, it is usually in the lower extremities because veins there get the most vigorous workout. Leg veins, in particular, are under stress because they bear the brunt of the body's weight. In

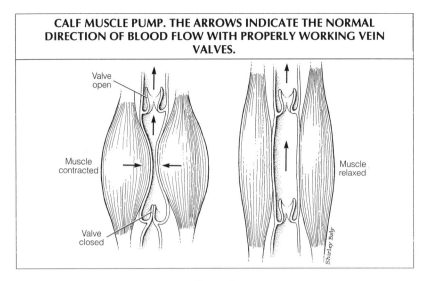

CALF MUSCLE PUMP. THE ARROWS INDICATE THE NORMAL DIRECTION OF BLOOD FLOW WITH PROPERLY WORKING VEIN VALVES.

Figure 6

addition, venous blood in the lower extremities must move uphill against the flow of gravity. Imagine how much pressure your leg veins would need to endure in order to get blood to rise nearly five feet if they didn't have vein valves to help spread the workload!

Vein valves can fail in many ways. For example, when abnormal pressure is put on a deep vein (as the result of injury, obesity or extensive exercise), the muscles that surround the deep vein keep it from getting out of shape. Veins must keep their shape because when they become too wide, for example, the valves will not meet anymore and there is nothing to direct the blood in an upward direction. Then when you stand still, or sit still, the blood effectively flows backward and just settles or pools in your leg veins.

In the normal leg, blood flows toward the heart and away from the saphenous and other, unnamed superficial veins to the deep veins. Valves in perforator veins control the direction of this inward flow and prevent blood from going backward from deep veins to the saphenous veins. In healthy legs, all systems are geared to take the load off the unprotected saphenous veins.

A harmful chain reaction can start when blood flows in the wrong direction (going, for example, from the deep to saphenous veins or pooling in the saphenous veins). The extra load on the saphenous vein causes it to dilate, stretch and widen. When this happens, more valves within the saphenous vein malfunction and a longer column of blood must be supported by the remaining valves and vein walls.

Saphenous veins, which carry about 10% of the venous blood back to the heart, can lose their shape more easily than deep veins because they are not protected and supported by muscle and tough fibrous tissue like deep veins. When someone develops a vein problem, it is almost always in the saphenous veins and their tributaries. Sometimes perforator veins can prevent saphenous veins from becoming varicose by relieving pressure in them. Perforator veins become an escape route by shifting the load to the stronger deep veins.

In general, the normal return of venous blood depends on the heart, the most powerful pump in the body, and on a remarkable "second heart," known as the venous muscle pump.

The venous muscle pump is a complex muscle action applied to the deep veins of the legs every time the legs move. Acting as a peripheral heart, the venous muscle pump is actually a number of separate but well integrated muscle groups surrounding the deep veins of the leg and thigh.

There are actually four separate pumps in the leg: one in the foot just below the ankle, the others in the calf, thigh and abdomen. Venous blood travels from capillaries to venules (tiny veins) to larger veins. From the ankle upward, venous blood flows from the saphenous to deep veins via perforator veins. As the deep veins are squeezed or compressed by the muscles that surround them, the blood is pumped into the femoral vein at the groin and then finally to the heart. When you walk, the peripheral pump is activated into returning a greatly increased volume of blood toward the heart—considerably more than when you are at rest.

Many believe the pump in the calf is the most efficient venous pump because your calf has three deep veins encompassed by muscles that squeeze the veins much more rigorously than muscles in the thigh or abdomen. Each muscle contraction in the calf can generate as much as 120 mm of mercury squeezing the deep veins and forcing venous flow upwards toward the heart.

It seems like a perfect system, yet it fails in almost half of the American people by the time they reach the fifth decade of their lives. The next chapter looks at what goes wrong, the different kinds of problems that arise along with their reasons, and possible ways to deal with them.

Notes

For basic references on the circulatory system and the anatomy of leg veins, we consulted two fine medical textbooks: *The Pathology and Surgery of the Veins of the Lower Limb* by Harold Dodd and Frank B. Cockett (Chapters 3 and 4) and *Sclerotherapy: Treatment of Varicose and Telangiectatic Leg Veins* by Mitchel P. Goldman (Chapter 1).

Other useful articles: "The Saphenous Valves in Varicose Veins" by Jesse Edwards and Edward Edwards in the *American Heart Journal,* 1940; and "Varicose Veins: Gross Anatomy and Development" by L.T. Cotton in *The British Journal of Surgery.*

CHAPTER 2

■■■■■■■■■■■■■■■■■■■■■■■■■■■■■

THE SYMPTOMS

A varicose vein is simply a vein in which the valves don't work. When the valves don't work, pressure builds up inside the vein and the vein becomes dilated, stretched and tortuous. The reasons the valves malfunction will be discussed in the next chapter.

The symptoms for varicose veins vary. They can include any of the following:

1. The presence of twisted, bulging blue lines running down part or all of a leg;
2. Legs that ache or become painful or tired and weak, especially after long periods of sitting or standing;
3. Restless legs, or legs that are so uncomfortable that a person has difficulty standing on both feet at once;
4. Burning or itchy skin on the legs; and
5. Legs and/or ankles that become swollen and possibly have a brownish pigmentation or other unsightliness.

Sometimes my patients will have just one of these symptoms. More often, they present multiple symptoms, as in the case of Mary N., a 44-year-old teacher who, before she was treated, experienced "pain, aches, throbbing and stinging . . . particularly severe in my ankles and thighs. I had trouble standing on both feet and constantly shifted my weight from one foot to the other. The pain in my legs sometimes kept me awake at night."

Of these symptoms, the most common is dull aching or tiredness and a feeling of fullness in the limb after prolonged periods of standing upright or sitting. That's when night cramps, or charley horse, in the calf muscles are likely to be a complaint. These symptoms all become worse toward the end of a busy day or during menstruation.

You might think that someone standing all day *should* have tired legs. Does this necessarily mean the person has varicose veins? The answer is no. However, the condition could be symptomatic of varicose veins if:

1. The aching becomes so intense and happens with such regularity that you limit your activities to avoid the pain; and
2. The aching gets worse even though you have done nothing extraordinary, like a 10-mile uphill hike, to aggravate the problem.

People have different levels of tolerance for the discomfort, pain or cosmetic disfigurement of varicose veins. Many seek treatment just for cosmetic reasons. Most see a doctor when one or more symptoms bother them. Let's take a closer look at the three most common symptoms: aching, disfigurement and swelling.

ACHING: In general, *any* aching or feeling of tiredness in the legs brought on by prolonged standing or prolonged sitting and relieved by leg elevation is due to varicose veins—unless proven otherwise. The problem is failed or incompetent valves in the saphenous and/or perforator veins, causing the blood to pool or flow the wrong way. The best that can be said about the ache associated with varicose veins is that it is almost never a true pain. It is generally described as a feeling of heaviness or fatigue in the legs, a dull ache. These discomforts can rarely be pinpointed, but when the ache is localized, it is generally over a varicose vein or a cluster of them.

When someone is suffering with varicose veins, it is usually aching legs that prompt him or her to seek a doctor's help, and it is a symptom that is easy to treat, at least temporarily. The two diametrically opposed solutions are rest and exercise. Lying down with your legs elevated above the level of your heart will bring relief by using gravity to solve the problem, but walking, running or dancing will also help you feel better. But iron shirts, wait on line at the supermarket, spend an evening at a cocktail party or fly across the continent and your legs will probably suffer. Movement helps because it exercises leg muscles that surround the deep veins, making them work more efficiently. When the deep veins are more efficient, surface veins can empty into them via the perforator veins. The problem causing the ache or tired feeling is temporarily solved.

However, if you have a sharp or sudden acute pain, see a doctor. It could be the beginning of a dangerous disease of the arteries or another serious problem. Also, if your leg pain gets worse with exercise, you might not have varicose veins. You could have a condition such as hardening of the arteries, a vascular disease which, if not treated, could have serious consequences. Or your problem could be fairly simple, like a pulled muscle resulting from an inadequate warm-up before exercises. Give it some thought. If you don't think the pain resulted from exercising, and more exercising makes it worse, do not guess: see a doctor.

DISFIGUREMENT: This is the most obvious sign of varicose veins and the one that most people associate with the condition. The disfigurement, usually progressive, often begins with the appearance of a small cluster of tortuous or snake-like veins. This cluster of varicosities can occur alone or become part of a larger problem that affects the entire saphenous system of veins. When that happens these veins become progressively bunched, twisted, lumped and contorted until they are angry, blue and bulging.

Perhaps your legs don't look that bad—just bad enough. You have some clusters of spider veins and some prominent blue lines. Spider veins are not true varicose veins, although they are often associated with varicose veins. So you're wondering if you have varicose veins.

One way to determine this is to put your feet up and see what happens. Ordinarily, when a person with a healthy leg stands, veins in the lower limb will bulge slightly. This bulging disappears when the person lies down or elevates the legs. A varicose vein generally will not disappear completely when the leg is changed from the upright to the prone position, because the faulty vein has stretched beyond its normal diameter and length. The varicose vein continues to be abnormally twisted and tortuous.

The extent of the problem, and even more important the symptoms, seldom corresponds to the number or size of protruding leg veins. Legs with varicose veins can look quite different. Obvious and bulging varicosities—especially in men—frequently are present with few symptoms. Conversely, some women with few visible varicosities often have severe pain or other symptoms. Women hide varicose veins better than men because women have a thicker layer of fat under the skin. Varicose veins are more noticeable in women with slender legs; women with heavier legs may have a pretty advanced case of varicose veins and show nothing at all on the surface. However, generalizations like these don't tell the whole story. The look, size and number of varicosities and the symptoms of varicose veins vary from one individual to the next.

One woman's varicose veins may be invisible in her thigh. Another may have an occasional vein popping up just underneath the skin. The calf of a third woman may have masses of veins that stand out as twisted blue cords, causing ridges or corrugations in the skin. A fourth could have only a few small spider veins with no other visible evidence of the varicose veins that cause so much pain.

Fads and fashion have a lot to do with the extent to which people rush to doctors to get help with varicose veins. Varicosities that disfigure the leg are no problem in floor-length dresses or pantsuits, but tennis outfits and rising hemlines provide opportunities for vascular surgeons to do a lot of work. With the current popularity of outdoor aerobic sports, more men also are worrying about their varicose veins than in past years. Chapter 4 has an extensive discussion of how to treat varicose veins. It should be noted here, however, that elevating your legs or getting more leg exercise (the temporary solutions already mentioned for aching legs) will not erase blue lines and bulges. The treatment for varicose veins depends on the extent of the problem. Often, when a few small varicosities begin to show, they turn out to be a minor problem. The doctor may find no sign that the greater saphenous vein is involved. Patients in this group are often relieved to learn that surgery is not needed. Surgery is recommended when the problem becomes so severe that it interferes with the quality of life, when it leads to complications or when a complication already exists.

Some patients will request "injections" as a cosmetic cure or to relieve discomfort. This technique, called sclerotherapy, requires a doctor to inject a corrosive chemical at various points along the varicose vein in order to "plug" the vein by forming a clot. This reroutes the blood through other, hopefully normal veins. This results in the disappearance of the unsightly varicosity. Sclerotherapy is safe, but it has some drawbacks, which are discussed in detail in Chapter 4: After three years, sclerotherapy fails in 60%–70% of all cases and the patient is left with the same old problem to cure.

One final thought on disfigurement: Not all blue lines running down a leg are varicose veins. In some, especially fair skinned people, a blue line running down the leg could be a prominent but harmless healthy vein. However, in others it could be a hint of trouble to come, particularly for those men and women whose mothers or grandmothers had varicose veins.

SWELLING: When varicose veins are involved, ankle swelling is fairly common. It generally shows up at the end of the day and especially affects people with standing occupations, including salespersons, bartenders, waitresses, security guards, dentists and surgeons. However, swollen ankles, legs and feet are not a sure sign of varicose veins. Such swelling can be triggered by a number of things. Anyone who spends hours standing, or sitting with the knees bent, can develop swollen legs. Even shoes or socks that are too tight can cause swelling.

A swollen leg is a challenge to the doctor who must rule out many other causes before telling you the swelling is due to varicose veins. Your doctor might try to determine if you have a blood clot in one of the leg's deep veins, heart failure, too few red blood cells (anemia), too little protein in the blood or a condition called lymphedema, which is a disorder that results in a swelling of the lower extremities and is caused by high venous pressure in the legs. Expect your doctor to run some tests if you have a swollen leg. The methods used to diagnose varicose veins are discussed in Chapter 4.

Don't ignore swollen legs or ankles. The potential causes are serious if left untreated. If varicose veins are causing your limbs to swell, surgery will probably be the recommended course of action.

Varicose veins have symptoms besides aching, disfigurement and swelling. These findings include itching, discoloration or pigmentation of the skin, night cramps and skin that seems to grow thin and shine. For example, the skin over the area of a varicose vein can be discolored with a light brown or blue tint. The discoloration is caused by a hemorrhage under the skin or chronic infections brought about by phlebitis (a common complication of varicose veins that is discussed in Chapter 6). The treatment and causes of these symptoms vary.

Another symptom is a night cramp or so called charley horse. These very painful muscle spasms occur most frequently in the calf at night or when you are asleep and are a common symptom associated with varicose veins. They often show up in patients with varicose veins after they have had long periods of standing without any other exercise. For some people, they are the earliest symptom. However, others with varicose veins never experience a night cramp. After 4,000 years of suffering with them, we still do not know what causes charley horse. One treatment is a gentle massage, followed by walking. Another solution: Quinamm, a prescription drug containing quinine.

Varicose veins can have more serious complications, including hemorrhaging, blood clots, phlebitis, swollen ankles and leg ulcers. The symptoms for these complications vary but they tend to be intense. Sometimes patients will experience sudden, debilitating pain and a feeling of weakness accompanied by fever, chills and a loss of appetite. Others will experience tenderness in their calves and an area of inflammation in the lower leg. Some will see a blush color around the ankle where the skin feels wooden to the touch. Sometimes the legs can turn blue, or even several shades paler accompanied by pain in the groin and thigh. These are signs that the patient has one of the complications that come with varicose veins. A detailed discussion of these complications, their symptoms, causes and treatment appears in Chapter 6.

Not all leg symptoms are due to varicose veins. People can have relatively symptomless varicosities, but they also can suffer with discomfort in the legs because of an arterial disorder, flat feet, arthritic knees or a back ailment. In fact, all symptoms of varicose veins may have other causes. So if you experience any of them, visit your doctor.

Unfortunately for you and your doctor, the symptoms of varicose veins do not necessarily correspond to the seriousness of the disorder. They have more to do with the patient's circulation, good or bad. Someone who has several circulatory problems in the venous system, such as multiple malfunctioning vein valves, will tend to suffer more with the symptoms of varicose veins than someone whose circulatory problems are more limited. Not everyone with varicose veins experiences the same degree of pain and discomfort.

Notes

The textbooks cited after Chapter 1 are two good sources for descriptions of the symptoms of varicose veins and their complications. In the

Dodd and Cockett book, Chapter 6 deals with symptoms described throughout this chapter. In Goldman's book, see Chapter 2.

An excellent article on this subject of how to recognize the symptoms of varicose veins appeared in the journal, *Postgraduate Medicine,* entitled "Varicose Veins: Their symptoms, complications and management" by Karl Lofgren. (June 1979)

CHAPTER 3

■■■■■■■■■■■■■■■■■■■■■■■■■■■■■■■■■■■

THE CAUSES

No one knows why varicose veins develop. The term describes a condition, not a clearly understood process: A varicose vein is one in which the valves no longer work properly, causing blood to flow the wrong way and pool in veins that become dilated and tortuous.

That definition implies that faulty valves cause varicose veins, but many doctors believe that malfunctioning valves are part of the problem and not necessarily the *cause* of the problem. Scientists continue to debate theories about the causes of varicose veins.

To find some answers, consider the following clues:

1. Varicose veins are almost always found in the legs, suggesting that the condition is brought on, or at least aggravated, by a human's upright position.
2. The incidence increases with age, suggesting that it is a condition that takes many years to develop and could be influenced by lifestyle (e.g., diet and exercise).
3. By some estimates, four times as many women as men have varicose veins, suggesting that female hormones might be a contributing factor.
4. Varicose veins are virtually unknown in undeveloped or emerging countries; however, as soon as these nations become industrialized, the incidence increases. This finding suggests that lifestyle plays a role in causing varicose veins.

As tantalizing as those clues are, they don't tell us the causes that doctors need to know to treat varicose veins effectively, and someday even prevent them.

The scientific debate now seems focused on a chicken-or-egg dilemma: Do varicose veins begin in the walls of your veins when

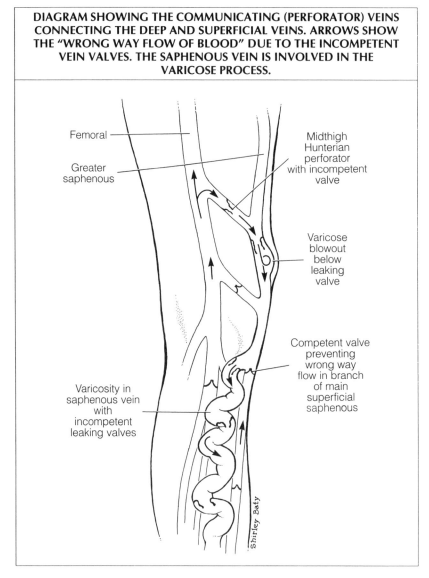

DIAGRAM SHOWING THE COMMUNICATING (PERFORATOR) VEINS CONNECTING THE DEEP AND SUPERFICIAL VEINS. ARROWS SHOW THE "WRONG WAY FLOW OF BLOOD" DUE TO THE INCOMPETENT VEIN VALVES. THE SAPHENOUS VEIN IS INVOLVED IN THE VARICOSE PROCESS.

Femoral

Greater saphenous

Midthigh Hunterian perforator with incompetent valve

Varicose blowout below leaking valve

Competent valve preventing wrong way flow in branch of main superficial saphenous

Varicosity in saphenous vein with incompetent leaking valves

Shirley Baty

Figure 7

they stretch and dilate, causing the valves to malfunction, or do the valves malfunction first, causing the veins' walls to stretch? Currently, there are six prevailing theories: the malfunctioning vein valve; the weak vein wall; heredity; the A-V shunt; a low-fiber diet; and the "educational blues."

Each could be a primary cause or a contributing factor. It is possible, for example, that only half the people in the world are born with a tendency toward varicose veins and varicosities develop only if certain other factors are present.

The Malfunctioning Valve

This theory says that malfunctioning or incompetent valves are the starting point from which varicose veins develop. It implies that there is no inherent defect in the vein walls or the valves per se. Rather, you have an absence or shortage of valves in your saphenous and/or perforator veins, and/or your valves just deteriorate with age. The theory relies on the notion that man's erect posture overloads the valves by putting too much pressure on veins in the lower extremities.

This overload, combined with a shortage of valves, or a malfunctioning valve, will cause one of the valves to fail. This failed valve then increases the amount of pressure on your vein wall below. When that vein wall stretches, it pulls open the doors on the next, lower set of valves, in turn putting abnormal pressure on the vein wall below that, and so on, until all of your valves fail like a set of dominoes. As a result, the blood pools so much that leg veins become stretched, twisted, lumpy and visible under the skin.

William Harvey was the first to call attention to vein valves in Padua, Italy in 1628. His valve theory was debated for many years before it was finally accepted by many in the medical community. Since then, many doctors have refreshed and expanded his work on the function of vein valves, notably John Ludbrook in 1966.

The evidence for the domino theory is largely empirical, based on the anatomical study of live patients and not-so-live cadavers and on deductive logic.

Relying on their own experience with many patients, vascular specialists generally agree that the more functioning valves you have, the less chance you have of getting varicose veins. As stated earlier, one study reported that people with a normal greater saphenous vein have valves every 3.5 inches compared to one in every 6.5 inches for those with varicosities. Other studies suggest that the number of vein valves you have is genetically determined.

Vascular surgeons have found, for example, that families with a strong hereditary predisposition to varicose veins tend to have valves missing just below the point where the greater saphenous and femoral veins meet.

Some doctors, however, reject the incompetent valve theory. Dr. Sidney Rose of the University Hospital of South Manchester in England argues that it "is presumptive rather than proven" and says "there is a good deal of argument against it." He says, for example, that leg veins function well when they are used as a substitute for arteries in heart bypass operations. Even though they are exposed to much greater pressure when used this way, the vein walls tend to get bulkier or thicker after bypass surgery; they do not stretch out of shape as the incompetent valve theory would suggest.

Rose also says valves have withstood attempts to rupture them at well over 300 mm of mercury pressure. (In contrast, as noted before, the normal arterial blood pressure in your arm could be 120 mm Hg.) Perhaps most importantly, he says varicosities are routinely found below normal valves. And vice versa: It's not uncommon to see that only part of the vein is stretched out of shape below a malfunctioning valve. Ultimately, Rose argues that varicose veins are caused by weak spots in the vein walls, not by malfunctioning valves.

Weak Walls

This theory states that varicose veins are caused by weak vein walls that stretch when exposed to undue pressure. When the walls stretch, your vein gets a distorted shape that makes it impossible for your valves to work properly because the valve rings (which are embedded in vein walls around each valve) also get stretched in the process. Why do some people have weak vein walls? One answer revolves around hormones.

It is fairly common for pregnant women to get varicose veins. They particularly show up in the second and successive pregnancies. Doctors used to think pregnant women got varicose veins because they had a greater volume of blood flowing through their circulatory systems and this, combined with the expansion of the uterus, put added pressure on the leg veins. Now, however, scientists know that varicosities appear in women very early in their pregnancies, before the uterus and blood volume expand. Sometimes, the very first sign of a pregnancy is the onset of painful legs accompanied with the sudden appearance of a cluster of varicosities. Scientists believe these clusters occur because of the surge of hormones that women get as soon as they become pregnant. Those hormones soften the collagen fibers in the uterus and pelvic ligaments (giving babies room to grow).

Vein walls also have collagen fibers, as well as muscles and elastic tissue. Proponents of the weak wall theory argue that a surge of estrogen will affect vein walls as well as the uterus. This same hormonal surge occurs just before and during menstruation, which is also when women complain of aching legs and other varicose-like symptoms.

It has been noted before that women are far more prone to varicose veins than men. The hormonal changes may explain the difference between the sexes. However, what about men? And what about women who have never been pregnant? They get varicose veins, too, but they don't experience the surge of hormones related to pregnancy.

Some scientists believe their problems can be explained by the genes they inherited. Vein walls for some men and women are weak because of an inherited genetic defect that upsets the balance of muscle, collagen and fibrous cells in their vein walls. This imbalance makes the muscles and elastic tissue in the veins unable to contract after they are exposed to a surge of pressure.

In effect, then, their vein walls are like cheap balloons; if you blow them up and let the air out, they never quite regain their old taut shape. Once the walls are stretched, they stay stretched, and so do the valve rings; the valves themselves then wither away from disuse.

Dr. Sidney Rose argues that the weak wall theory explains many things, including the way some people can have so-called blowouts in their veins without having any malfunctioning valves nearby.

Heredity

Some scientists believe that weak valves, a shortage of valves or a tendency toward weak vein walls have only one explanation: defective genes.

In my experience, more than 75% of those who have varicose veins also have other immediate family members, especially their mothers or grandmothers, with a history of varicosities. Researchers have found that mothers and daughters often have an identical pattern of varicosities. Some scientists have found that children whose parents had varicose veins are twice as likely to have a malfunctioning saphenofemoral valve (where the femoral vein connects with the saphenous vein in the groin).

This genetic tendency seems to affect broad groups of people. For example, the Irish have a higher rate of varicose veins than the Scots, who in turn have a higher rate than the English, according to some studies. Researchers, particularly Denis Burkitt, who spent many years as a missionary physician in Africa before devoting his time to international medical research, also have found that African blacks, Nilo-Hamitics, Arabic races, natives of India and the Australian aborigines are all peoples virtually free of varicose veins and the associated problems. However, American blacks suffer varicose veins at the same rate as the American white population. Is this because a number of American blacks carry a trace of white blood or is it because they share the same culture? We simply do not know.

The Arterio-Venous Connection or A-V Shunts

You recall from Chapter 1 that veins and arteries are separated at one end of the circulatory system by the heart and at the other end by capillaries. The heart takes blood from the veins, refuels it, and sends it back to the rest of the body through the arteries.

The critical role played by the capillaries is to act as nature's miniature pressure valves. The capillaries keep the enormous pressure of the arteries from overwhelming the veins whose walls are weaker than arterial walls. Capillaries also make sure that arterial blood feeds tissues with oxygen and other nutrients.

Sometimes, however, an accident of nature will cause arterial blood to bypass the capillaries through an arterio-venous, or A-V, shunt. When normally dormant A-V shunts are activated (for reasons yet unknown), your blood effectively turns a corner at much greater speed and at higher, pulsating pressure, which can damage the veins, causing varicosities. Think of a racing car turning a corner at the Indy 500 with only a slight touch of the brake. Presumably, the car would crash into the side of the track, or at least bang into a wall before careening onward.

Remember that normal blood pressure in the branchial *artery* of your arm could be about 120mm of mercury pressure compared to only 8 mm of pressure in a *vein* in that same arm. Similar differences in blood pressures exist in the main veins and arteries of your legs. With A-V shunts, the arteries and veins are connected through the arterioles and venules, the narrowest parts of the arterial and venous systems. The narrow shunts act as something of a brake, but they are not as good as a network of capillaries.

The A-V shunt theory was proposed in 1953 by two Spanish researchers, Piulachs and Vidal-Barraquer. They noticed that some patients with varicose veins had problems outside the normal saphenous route while others had nothing wrong with their valves. After investigating, they concluded that these A-V shunts are present in all people, in various size and numbers, and all types of varicosities result from them.

What causes A-V shunts to activate? Three possible answers have been offered: accidents, disease and hormones. A traumatic accident that leaves tissue damaged can lead to the formation or reactivation of A-V shunts, as can an unidentified disease that causes a neurological imbalance of the autonomic nervous system. Hormones also get blamed because functioning A-V shunts are found during three periods of heightened hormonal activity—puberty, pregnancy and menopause.

The A-V shunt theory has received recent support from researchers like Dr. Henry Haimovici, clinical professor (emeritus) of surgery at Albert Einstein College of Medicine in New York. Haimovici reports that in most people, the first sign of varicose veins appears in the tributaries, not in the main saphenous or perforator veins where malfunctioning valves can be found at later stages of the disease. Haimovici also cites other research that I did with Dr. Sebastiano Cassaro, a colleague at the Cabrini Medical Center in New York City. We found that blood flowing through varicose veins has a much higher level of oxygen and other gases than blood flowing through healthy veins. The higher levels of oxygen are usually found in arteries. Therefore, our assumption is that some arterial blood is bypassing the capillaries (through an A-V shunt) before getting into varicose veins.

This and other research done with the latest diagnostic equipment—like the Doppler probe mentioned in Chapter 4 and venograms which are X rays of the veins performed after a dye is injected into them—all support the notion of A-V shunts as the cause of the problem, he says.

Haimovici argues that this is why surgeons now more frequently operate on the tributaries and break the microscopic A-V shunts, in addition to removing the saphenous trunk when treating someone in the early stages of varicose disease.

The Low-Fiber Diet

So far, we've discussed four possible causes of varicose veins: malfunctioning valves, weak vein walls, heredity and A-V shunts. They all have one thing in common—the notion that there is little you can do to prevent varicose veins. Two other theories suggest you do have some power to prevent varicose veins, either by changing your diet to include more fiber or by being more active physically—or both.

The low-fiber diet theory is relatively simple: Your colon is attached to the lower spine and hangs like a punching bag. In animals walking on all fours, the colon swings freely. However, in humans, it hangs down, pressing and compressing the major veins of the trunk and lower abdomen against the bony spine. Those who have high-fiber diets empty their colons within an average of 35 hours after consuming a meal while those with low-fiber take 77 hours. A heavy colon (one filled with hard fecal matter) compresses veins more than an empty colon, and the more pressure on veins in the lower trunk, the harder the veins in the legs must work to drive blood past this point back to the heart. The harder the leg veins work, the more pressure there is on them, causing a tendency to develop varicose veins.

Doctors will tell you that some chronic constipation is caused by low-fiber diets, common in the Western Hemisphere (where, as previously noted, varicose veins also are most common). A low-fiber diet forces a person to strain to pass a stool and this straining puts great pressure on the abdominal muscles. Thomas Cleave, a surgeon in the British Royal Navy who pioneered this idea, argues that pressure from straining is passed to your leg veins, causing them to dilate. This dilation in turn separates the doors, or valve leaflets, on your valves and makes your valves malfunction.

Cleave's work has been supported by other prominent British physicians, including H.C. Trowell and Denis P. Burkitt. Burkitt noted that varicose veins are relatively rare in Africa. He suggests that this could be because the typical tribesman squats to pass a stool that is almost liquid. He notes the average American sits to defecate and passes a much harder stool. Burkitt's observation fits another part of the theory: that straining increases pressure on leg veins because it puts more pressure on a critical venous valve in the groin.

Remember: Long leg veins end in the pelvic area of the trunk. Researchers feel that tensing abdominal muscles by straining to pass a stool can damage the vein valves at the point where the lower limb veins join the veins in the trunk. Now recall the incompetent valve theory: Once the uppermost set of valves is damaged, it increases pressure on the next set down, and so on, as gravity does its work.

Fiber works by filling the colon with bulky roughage. A colon filled with roughage is light and stool passes from it quickly—often a full day earlier than stool with little roughage. Fiber is abundant in foods like raw fruits and vegetables, beans and peas, nuts and unprocessed sugar and grains. Foods with no fiber include processed sugar, meat, fish, eggs, fats, cheese, alchohol and milk. Some Third World peoples get their fiber by eating unprocessed grains and by chewing on sugarcane, spitting out the residue, but swallowing plenty of fiber in the process.

The low-fiber theory is supported by studies that have found a significant statistical correlation between varicose veins and diverticulitis, an illness in which sacs on the wall of the large bowel become inflamed. Diverticulitis is believed to be caused by constipation.

The theory makes sense, but it is not foolproof. The Masai, who live in southern Kenya and northern Tanzania, have virtually no venous disease or varicose veins, and they have a high fiber diet. However, they also suffer from serious constipation; it accounts for 27% of hospital admissions. This would seem to dispel the theory that constipation alone is a serious cause of varicose veins.

Educational Blues

Are you standing while reading this chapter? Probably not; you are probably sitting somewhere—on a bench, the sofa or a chair. These furniture pieces are as much a part of Western culture as bad diets, and some suspect just as much of a culprit in causing varicose veins.

Doctors agree that sitting on a chair does more damage to the circulation in your legs than sitting on the ground. How? One of the biggest challenges to leg veins is the force of gravity, which makes them work hard to return blood to the heart. Blood moves out of the leg when muscles squeeze the veins and push the blood upward.

When you're sitting in a chair, your legs don't move much and don't give gravity much of a challenge. Your legs below the knees are pointed straight down. Just think of how your feet and ankles swell on long plane or car rides. When you sit, you are letting gravity win. You also are putting unremitting pressure on the back of your thighs. This pressure compresses the veins. When you are sitting in a chair, the amount of stress on the walls of your saphenous and perforator veins **doubles**. Sitting increases pressure in your ankles, where the saphenous veins begin, by about 250%.

The theory was proposed as long ago as 1913, when Miyauchi, a doctor in Japan, noted that varicose veins were rare among the Japanese who at that time stayed in their homeland and followed the custom of eating while seated on the floor. He noticed that varicosities are more common among Japanese who emigrate to the West and adopt a life style that includes sitting in chairs. Now that the Japanese have adopted more Western ways at home and work (which means more sitting in chairs), it's not clear whether that has resulted in more incidents of varicose veins. However, since Miyauchi's 1913 study, other researchers have found a similar phenomenon: the virtual absence of varicose veins in cultures where chairs are fairly rare.

The good part of this research is that it provides a fairly simple, possible preventative remedy: avoid chairs as much as possible. However, it's obviously not that easy.

Just think for a minute how much you sit. You start in a high chair and then progress to sitting with your hands folded in kindergarten. You sit through elementary and high school, in college and perhaps at a white collar job until you retire to the South to sit in the sun. By the time you have earned a college degree, you have sat in a classroom on chairs for an average of five hours a day, five days a week, 10 months a year for 17 years. That's about 17,000 hours of sitting! Add three more hours a day of doing homework and three more of watching television and you have 28,000 hours.

The problem has intensified in recent decades as the American work force has moved from manufacturing jobs that require more frequent, full body movement, to service sector jobs, which are more sedentary. The impact is seen in a 1972 U.S. Public Health Service survey that reported that over 33% of all people in the U.S. had varicose veins and three million of them were under the age of 45.

Changing your lifestyle and work environment is difficult but not impossible. A high fiber diet and more exercise won't cure varicose veins once they show up, but they can help alleviate symptoms in mild cases and delay the onset of symptoms in others. People with more advanced cases of varicose veins need more aggressive treatment, the subject of Chapter 5.

First, let's take a quick look at what to expect when your doctor tests you for varicose veins.

Notes

The most extensive studies ever done on who gets varicose veins and when they get them were conducted in Switzerland throughout the 1970s. There, doctors looked at the medical histories of thousands of European people and concluded that varicose veins are found more in people as they reach middle age, more in women than in men and more in people from northern Europe than the Mediteranean. (One source is *Basle Study III* by L.K. Widmer, published by Hans Huber Publishers in 1978. Also, for a closer look at the influence of pregnancy, prolonged standing, tight garters and obesity, see "Causative Factors of Varicose Veins: Myths and Facts" by E. Guberan, L.K. Widmer, L. Glaus, R. Muller, A. Rougemont, A. DaSilva and F. Gendre in *VASA*, 1973.)

For more on Thomas L. Cleave's work, see his book *On Causation of Varicose Veins* (published 1960 by John Wright & Sons Ltd. of Bristol, United Kingdom).

For more on malfunctioning valves, see "Valvular Defect in Primary Varicose Veins—Cause or Effect?" by John Ludbrook in *The Lancet*, December 1963.

For more on vein walls, see Sidney Rose's article in the *Journal of Cardiovascular Surgery* entitled "Some thoughts on the aetiology of varicose veins" (1986) and "Anatomic Observations on Causes of

Varicose Veins," which is Chapter 2 in *Investigation of Chronic Venous Insufficiency* (published 1993 by Med-Orion Publishing in London and edited by J. Hobbs and A.N. Nicolaides).

Rose's theory is supported by a new study published in *Surgery* in April 1992, "Venous wall function in the pathogenesis of varicose veins" by G. Heather Clarke, S.N. Vasdekis, J.T. Hobbs and A.N. Nicolaides.

For discussions on the role of genes and heredity in getting varicose veins, see "Hereditary Factors in Venous Insufficiency" by Jorgen Gundersen and Mogens Hauge in *Angiology* (1969); "Lower Limb Venous Dynamics in Normal Persons and Children of Patients with Varicose Veins" by Brian Regan and Roland Folse in *Surgery, Gynecology and Obstetrics* (1971); "A Contribution to the Problem of the Inheritance of Primary Varicose Veins" by V. Matousek and I. Prerovsky in *Human Heredity* (1974); and "Importance of the Familial Factor in Varicose Disease" by Andre Cornu-Thenard, Pierre Boivin, Jean-Michel Baud, Isabelle DeVincenzi and Patrick Carpentier in the *Journal of Dermatology, Surgery and Oncology* (1994).

Henry Haimovici discusses Arterio-Venous shunts in "A new look at the pathogenesis and treatment of primary varicose veins" in *Contemporary Surgery* (October 1988). A-V shunts also are the focus of a paper "The Role of Arteriovenous Shunts in the Pathogenesis of Varicose Veins" published in the *Journal of Vascular Surgery* (1986).

Denis Burkitt, a missionary surgeon in Africa, makes a powerful argument for diet as a cause of varicosities in "Varicose Veins: Facts and Fantasy" published in *Arch Surgery* (1976). When he died in 1993, the international medical journal *The Lancet* said his work drastically changed people's eating habits all over the Western World by getting them to eat more high fiber foods.

The theory that chair sitting is a culprit was advanced by Colin James Alexander in a 1972 article "Chair-sitting and Varicose Veins" in *The Lancet*.

CHAPTER 4

■ ■

DIAGNOSING VARICOSE VEINS

Varicose veins, like speed limits and traffic signals, are considered a nuisance, but if you ignore any of them, you can die. Last year, more than 100,000 Americans died from some complication of varicose veins. Hundreds of thousands more were disfigured or disabled by them, many with the leg ulcers that can result from untreated varicose veins. Karl Lofgren of the Mayo Clinic estimates that chronic venous disease accounts for as much as 10% of all hospital admissions in the U.S. The cost of treatment, not to mention the loss of productive work hours, is huge for a so-called nuisance disease. To determine which treatment is best for you, your doctor first must make sure your symptoms cannot be attributed to another disease such as arthritis, a lower back problem or some other disorder.

Your doctor will want to examine all systems in the involved limb—veins, arteries and nerves—and the rest of you. Varicose veins can be caused by other problems, such as an abdominal mass or phlebitis (an inflammation of the vein) or even pregnancy. After questioning you about your symptoms and taking a family history, your doctor will probably ask you to lie down and raise your leg to drain your veins by gravity. Then he will put pressure over the groin area and ask you to stand as he continues to press in that area. If, when he lets go, any of your superficial veins suddenly fill up and bulge out under the skin, it means that a critical valve at the junction of the saphenous and femoral veins has failed or has been missing from birth. Sometimes a doctor will perform this test by putting a tourniquet (a large rubber band) around your leg as you're lying down. When you stand, if the veins beneath the tourniquet fill up, you probably have a faulty valve. This test can be repeated several times with your doctor applying pressure at various points to determine a more precise location of your valve failure.

Doctors also can find defective valves by studying your blood flow with a Doppler ulstrasonic detector. A Doppler probe operates on the principle of a sound wave. As your doctor moves the probe with its smooth surface along your calf, a crystal inside the probe produces a sound wave. The sound wave then gets bounced back from objects (cells within your blood) moving inside your veins and arteries. This ultrasound wave is picked up by a sensitive microphone inside the probe and made audible.

A Doppler probe is usually applied to your calf first because that is where the valves are concentrated, but it also is used to detect vein valve incompetence along the saphenous vein in your groin at that critical point where the saphenous and femoral veins meet.

With the Doppler probe positioned over your veins, your doctor will ask you to take a deep breath, hold it, and while still holding your breath, bear down. The medical term for this procedure is the valsalva maneuver. The procedure increases pressure in your leg veins. When you finally exhale, there is increased blood flow. All of this activity is audible on the Doppler monitor. Normally, the blood in your veins sounds like a throbbing "whoosh" and makes this sound every time you breathe. When the valsalva maneuver is done on a healthy person without varicose veins, the blood flow stops momentarily because there is pressure on the veins and there is no sound heard on the Doppler. When the valsalva maneuver is done on someone who has varicose veins that have developed because of incompetent vein valves in the groin, the Doppler probe will pick up a steady "whoosh" that indicates that blood is leaking backward down the leg vein. The valsalva maneuver is usually most reliable when a doctor is trying to determine if the valves in the groin or upper thigh are malfunctioning. The Doppler probe can also help a doctor find incompetent valves further down the leg without using the valsalva maneuver.

Another diagnostic test being used more frequently is called photoplesthysmography. Also known as LRR (for light reflecting rheography), this test is simple, relatively inexpensive and like the Doppler probe, noninvasive. It works with infrared light that is measured and recorded on paper as a graph when it is reflected off red blood cells circulating through your body. An intense red light can show the presence of a clot within the deep or superficial leg veins. Incompetent vein valves show up with other readings on the graph.

Photoplesthysmography also can be used to rule out varicose veins. If a young patient with prominent leg veins asks a doctor to surgically remove the veins or perform sclerotherapy, the doctor might use LRR to measure how long it takes for the veins to refill after the patient has been reclining. If the refilling time is normal, surgery might not be the answer; the problem could be simply a case of prominent veins, but not varicose veins.

In the last six or seven years, some doctors also have started using a duplex color Doppler analysis to evaluate blood flow. It operates on the same principle as ultrasound machines used in fetal monitoring during pregnancy and gives the doctor a two-color view of the circulatory system: the veins are blue, the arteries red. First, the affected area is covered with a harmless jelly that produces an airtight connection between the probe and the skin; then a plastic scanner is rolled over your leg. When blood is backing up in a vein, it shows as a red mass invading blue turf. The problem with this diagnostic tool is that it sometimes gives false negatives: there's no red invading blue but the patient still has other symptoms that strongly suggest varicose veins. If the symptoms persist, doctors might then do a venogram.

A venogram or phlebogram is the most invasive diagnostic test that a doctor can perform on your veins. This test is considered the "Gold Standard" because it gives the most accurate picture of veins in your lower extremity and the underlying problem. It requires a trained radiologist in a hospital setting to inject a contrast material into the foot vein. The material is then traced by X rays as it moves up the veins in your lower extremities. Your doctor might simultaneously ask you to do a valsalva maneuver (inhale, bear down, exhale) to determine if you have an incompetent vein valve at the critical connection between the deep and superficial saphenous vein in your groin. A venogram can also pinpoint other incompetent vein valves in the deep venous system in your leg, often a cause of serious problems as you grow older.

Now that you've been examined thoroughly, your doctor is ready to make a diagnosis. If you have varicose veins, expect the doctor to describe the treatments discussed in the next chapter.

THE VENOGRAM DRAMATICALLY DEMONSTRATES BELOW-KNEE
VARICOSITIES IN THE GREATER SAPHENOUS VEIN. THE
COMMUNICATING VEINS CONNECTING THE DEEP AND
SUPERFICIAL VEINS HAVE INCOMPETENT VEIN VALVES AND ARE
ALSO INVOLVED IN THE VARICOSE PROCESS.

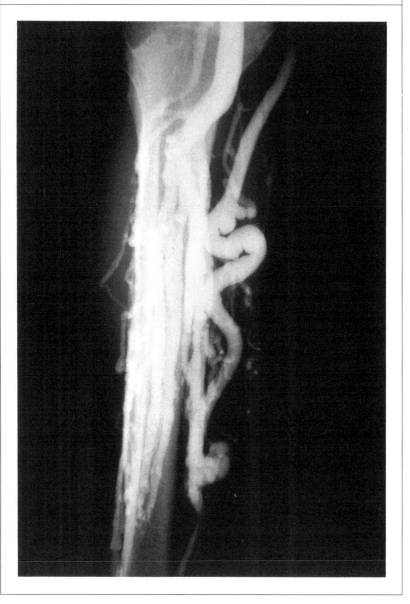

Figure 8

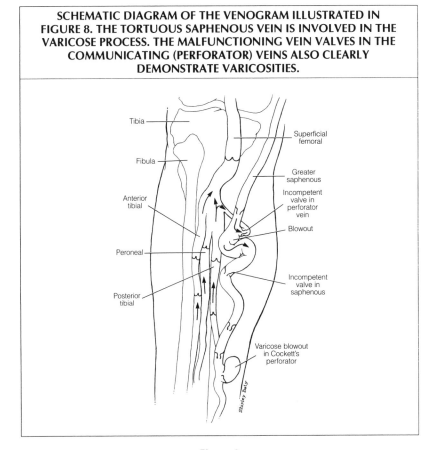

SCHEMATIC DIAGRAM OF THE VENOGRAM ILLUSTRATED IN FIGURE 8. THE TORTUOUS SAPHENOUS VEIN IS INVOLVED IN THE VARICOSE PROCESS. THE MALFUNCTIONING VEIN VALVES IN THE COMMUNICATING (PERFORATOR) VEINS ALSO CLEARLY DEMONSTRATE VARICOSITIES.

Figure 9

Notes

My own clinical experience of more than 25 years is the basis for this chapter.

For further reading, see the two medical textbooks cited after Chapter 1. Dodd and Cockett deal with diagnosing the problem in Chapter 7; Goldman does it in Chapter 5.

CHAPTER 5

■ ■

TREATING THE PROBLEM

Dr. Mitchel Goldman, a noted dermatologist in California who has written an excellent book on sclerotherapy, estimates that 80 million adults in the United States alone have varicose and spider veins. He believes that more than half who seek treatment do so not because they want to look better but because they want to feel better.

In treating varicose veins, doctors have three goals:

1. They want a cure, not a temporary fix;
2. They want to prevent complications that could have fatal consequences and/or treat any existing complications; and
3. They want to alleviate the cosmetic disfigurement often associated with varicose veins.

There are three basic ways to treat varicose veins: elastic stockings, injection therapy and surgery.

Which one is right for you? That depends on many things, including your age, your overall physical health and the extent and location of your varicosities. For example, if you are 90 and bedridden with a heart condition, it is unlikely that any doctor will recommend surgery to remove varicose veins. If you are a 35-year-old pregnant traffic cop whose varicose legs ache unbearably because your job requires you to stand all day, surgery also could be ruled out in favor of elastic stockings and/or bed rest as a temporary treatment for a temporary problem caused by the pregnancy. Surgery could be recommended, however, if you are an otherwise healthy individual whose varicose veins are due to malfunctioning valves or a weak or dilated vein wall in your saphenous veins.

To determine the best treatment for you, your doctor will perform or prescribe the tests described in the preceding chapter to make sure your symptoms cannot be attributed to another disease. In the process, your doctor will determine if your varicose veins are primary (i.e., occurred spontaneously) or secondary (i.e., triggered by some other ailment). The outcomes of these tests are important because they can indicate which treatment is best.

Following is a more detailed look at the three basic treatments.

Elastic Stockings

This treatment is called external compression therapy and it involves wearing specially fitted elastic stockings.

The stockings are designed to reduce edema, or swelling, in the lower extremities, thereby relieving some of the symptoms of varicose veins. By giving your saphenous and superficial veins more support, they also help increase the flow of blood in your legs back to your heart. An increased flow helps prevent stasis, or pooling, of blood in your varicosities, thus avoiding more serious complications discussed in the next chapter. Fitted elastic stockings are useful in some cases, but for most people they are not a satisfactory long term therapy. They are most helpful when surgery is impossible or undesirable, (for example, in the case of a pregnant woman or someone with chronic kidney or heart disease).

Elastic stockings have some drawbacks. First, they must fit properly or they will cause more discomfort than they will cure.

Your ankle and calf veins are under greater pressure, due to the laws of gravity. Your veins in this region need more support than those in your thighs. Modern fitted stockings are designed to apply a graduated pressure along the length of your leg. If a stocking does not fit properly, it could act as a tourniquet, squeezing your thigh veins even though it gives the proper compression to your calves and ankles. The fit is affected by the diameter of the stocking, the kind of elastic material used in it and its length.

Some patients require midthigh or leotard stockings, but most are prescribed stockings that cover the leg to just below the knee where most varicosities are concentrated. By supporting vein walls in superficial tissues, the stockings help increase the flow of blood returning to your heart and act in concert with the so-called "peripheral heart," the powerful calf muscle that pumps blood back up your leg as you walk.

Some stockings are custom fitted. These are the most expensive and most effective. Most are manufactured in ready-to-wear sizes that fit the majority of the population.

Second, stockings require a lot of education and strict compliance on the part of the wearers. They must wear them daily (no exceptions). The patient must pull them on before getting out of bed in the morning, and wear them throughout the work day no matter how uncomfortable they become. In the evening, after removing them, the wearer should elevate his or her legs for at least 30 minutes.

Obese people and the elderly often have trouble getting stockings on and off. Recognizing this, manufacturers have developed various aids. Some stockings are made with a zipper. Other patients depend on a slippery, parachute type of toeless stocking that they put on first; then they glide the elastic bandage over it; and finally, they pull the "parachute" out from underneath. Finally, to encourage compliance among fashion conscious patients, some manufactures produce elastic stockings in various colors.

All these devices help the patient follow the doctor's basic order: Wear those stockings without fail. However, compliance isn't complete unless patients remain on guard constantly to make sure that the stockings, that can be made of nylon and natural or synthetic rubber, don't lose their pressure. This is the biggest problem. The stockings stretch so gradually that the support needed can disappear and complications can occur before the patient realizes it.

The third disadvantage of elastic stockings is that they must be replaced periodically, generally every three months—and they are not cheap.

Knee-length stockings can cost $58 a pair, midthigh stockings $76 a pair and leotard models cost more, starting at $85 a pair. Some insurance carriers will reimburse only part of the entire amount on of the stockings and increasingly patients find that they have to pay for a greater portion of the cost themselves. Doctors usually recommend that the patient buy two new pairs at a time, so that one pair can be worn while the other is being washed. If the price never rises (which is extremely unlikely), knee-length stockings could cost you more than $360 a year. And you will bear this cost for the rest of your life!

The main reason that elastic stockings are not recommended for most people is that they are a short term solution to a long term problem. They do provide fair quick relief. Patients find the swelling and aching alleviated substantially, if not totally. In addition, sometimes they can shrink the varicosities and reduce ankle swelling or edema.

However, my patients generally have had the same experience as that reported by two famous vascular surgeons, John Bergan in San Diego and Norman Browse in London: If you stop using the stockings for any length of time, the varicosities and symptoms (aching, heaviness and swelling) return almost immediately. Sometimes they are worse than ever because varicose veins are progressive—they only get worse with time. Even pregnant women whose varicosities often disappear when they give birth find that they return later in life. These are the same varicosities that gave them trouble during their pregnancies and women who have varicose veins when they are pregnant can be pretty sure of seeing them reappear in their late 40s or 50s. You are usually stuck with varicose veins all your life unless you are cured, most often by surgery.

Injection Therapy

Also known as sclerotherapy, injection therapy requires your doctor to inject a corrosive chemical at various points into your varicose vein. Then he wraps your leg in an elastic bandage which MUST stay in place for a period, sometimes up to several weeks.

The chemical irritates the lining of your vein and causes a clot to form. The clot blocks blood from flowing in the wrong direction in your varicose vein and effectively forces venous blood to flow back up to the heart where it belongs. The effect is like having a highway patrol car sitting on the side of the road: It encourages you to obey the speed limit and other rules of the road, at least for a while.

The biggest problem with sclerotherapy is that the benefits are short-lived. The problems reappear in 60%–70% of all cases within three to four years if sclerotherapy is done on veins that really required surgery because the veins were too stretched out for the chemically induced clot to work. Generally, surgeons and dermatologists agree that for veins measuring three millimeters or less, sclerotherapy can be effective. Anything larger requires surgery.

Sclerotherapy can be a prolonged process that requires many visits to your doctor's office. During each visit, your doctor will make 6 to 10 injections in whatever leg is affected. Then he will apply an elastic bandage or a compressive dressing that must fit properly and be worn for varying periods, sometimes up to two weeks. At that point, you return to the doctor's office and repeat the process, which continues until all the varicosities have been injected.

The process sounds awful and it can hurt if saline is used. Other solutions hurt less, but whatever solution is used, sclerotherapy is a safe procedure. It is most successful when the problem is relatively minor, such as dilated superficial (or spider) veins or residual varicosities that are unsightly but not dangerous.

However, sclerotherapy also has some drawbacks. First, as noted above, the results are temporary. Unless sclerotherapy is done only on the tiniest veins and combined with surgical removal of the saphenous veins, the problem usually is back within three to four years.

Second, there is the possibility that the clot created to plug your vein will move and become hazardous by traveling to your heart, brain or lung. The clot could be dislodged if the patient did something as simple as remove the compression bandage and the result could be fatal. Normally, however, the clots do not move. They are effectively locked into place by the scar tissue that forms around them.

Third, sclerotherapy can cause pain and tenderness that can last for weeks when doctors inject saline, a salt solution that is designed to irritate the vein wall. Less painful alternatives to saline are available, like polidocanol, which was originally a local anesthetic.

Fourth, sclerotherapy can be counterproductive as a cosmetic cure because in some people it leaves patches of yellow-brown discolored skin at the site of the injection or along the vein. This stain, which occurs when the sclerosing fluid leaks into tissue around the vein, can be permanent.

Sclerotherapy is more popular in Europe, particularly Ireland and England where medicine is socialized and the governments have determined that this cheaper (albeit temporary) approach is better than surgery whenever possible. Doctors George Fegan of Dublin and John T. Hobbs of St. Mary's Hospital in London have reported excellent results with sclerotherapy. Fegan says he gets fewer side effects by injecting sodium tetradecyl, as opposed to other substances.

Hobbs, however, has observed that the treatment must be precise: injections must be made at exactly the right spots; pressure must be applied at the right points; and bandaging has to be done a certain way. If the needle hits a nerve, the pain is severe and can last for days. If too much of the chemical agent is injected, patients can get toxic reactions such as thirst, shivering, headaches and sometimes chest pains and upset stomachs. Sometimes an ulcer can occur at the injection site. And if the substance is accidentally injected into an artery, the foot can become gangrenous. English doctors will recommend surgery over sclerotherapy if a patient has sizeable varicose veins, or if the patient has very fat legs because it is more difficult to apply proper pressure with stockings or bandages to fat legs.

In the U.S., sclerotherapy is more likely to be recommended by general practitioners and dermatologists who are not trained in vascular surgery. Indeed, some patients in recent years have been lured to sclerotherapy by newspaper and other ads that billed the procedure as a *new* "microcure" that supposedly lasts longer than surgery and is free of scarring or risky side effects. The ads were placed by an Illinois-based firm called Vein Clinics of America; it sold franchises to doctors who trained nurses to give the injections. In 1994, the Federal Trade Commission chastised the company and it agreed to stop making what the FTC considered false claims. The franchises are still functioning all over the U.S.

Sclerotherapy has a proper place in the treatment of varicose veins, and American vascular specialists will more likely recommend sclerotherapy after larger varicosities are surgically removed. Then they can treat the residual, tiny varicosities. There is a need for sclerotherapy after surgery because that's when circulating blood finds new pathways, often using veins that were dormant before surgery. Sometimes this process results in new varicosities. When combined with a surgical "stripping" operation (described in detail next), injection therapy also is less extensive (requiring fewer than a half dozen injections) and most effective. One study in the United Kingdom found a 90% success rate after three to four years when sclerotherapy was combined with a surgical "stripping" operation.

Sclerotherapy also is used sometimes during a pregnancy when varicosities are severe but surgery is not an option. It is unclear what, if any, effect the chemical agent used in the process has on the fetus.

For this reason, sclerotherapy is not generally done on pregnant women except in the most dire circumstances.

Also, sclerotherapy is not recommended for those who are seriously overweight, that is, more than 25% above their recommended weight. The legs of obese people do not tolerate elastic bandages very well because the bandages tend to slip off the leg. The fat in the legs also makes the bandages ineffective because the pressure is never correctly applied. Thus, the problem often returns.

Surgery

Sooner or later, surgery is inevitable and the treatment of choice for most people because varicose veins are a progressive problem and the treatments already described are only quick solutions to a long term problem. For many people, surgery is frightening. However, it has one great advantage: When it's done, it's done. After surgery, you will feel better and look better, and your varicose veins will probably never bother you again. There is no guarantee that new varicose veins won't crop up, but they are tiny and rare.

The basic operation is simple. A vascular surgeon removes your saphenous veins—the veins that have the faulty valves—and thereby eliminates the major path that your blood has been using to fall back into your legs. Your blood is then forced to flow up to your heart through healthy veins with good, working valves.

Surgery can be recommended for four possible reasons: relief from the sometimes debilitating symptoms of varicose veins, prevention of complications, relief from complications and cosmesis (to make your legs look better). Surgery is not recommended if you have some temporary health problems like weeping dermatitis, acute skin infection, uncontrolled metabolic disease, pregnancy, anemia and poor general health. It also is not recommended if you have arterial insufficiency or chronic lymphedema or if you are very old.

You are your own best judge of whether it is necessary, but if the quality of your life suffers or your workday is interrupted by the symptoms and swelling that varicose veins can cause, surgery is probably your best option.

Before describing the operation, recuperation period and possible side effects, here is some information about the process of getting to the point where you are wheeled into an operating room:

1. Don't feel guilty about seeking a second opinion about the need for surgery. When doctors recommend surgery, they are, after all, stating their opinion, and they understand that another doctor may have a different view. To reduce unnecessary surgery, some health insurance plans now require second opinions and pay for them. However, the doctor who provides the second opinion does so as an impartial party and is prohibited by medical ethics from performing the surgery.

    You can get the names of vascular surgeons from your county Medical Society if your own doctor cannot provide them.

2. Except in very severe cases that require emergency treatment, surgery for varicose veins is elective, meaning you get in line behind others who also need an operating room and it may take weeks before your doctor can make a reservation for you at your local hospital. However, you can often make good use of the time before you are admitted by getting insurance and hospital paperwork, and the necessary lab work, completed.

    You can expect to go into the hospital early in the morning on the day of your operation and leave that afternoon. (Insurance companies no longer pay for a night's stay before or after the surgery. Some insurance companies refer to the pre-op night as an unnecessary "hotel" expense.)

3. Generally, your insurance policy will cover the full cost of hospitalization but not your doctor's entire fee. The surgeon's fee should be between $2,500 and $3,500 for one leg, double that amount for two, with fees slightly higher in the Northeast, Florida and California. In addition, you will have to pay an anesthesiologist's fee.

    Most good insurance policies will cover 80% of the fees charged by your surgeon and anesthesiologist, plus 100% of your hospital-related expenses.

On the day of your operation, most of your discussion with the anesthesiologist will focus on the choice of anesthesia. You can be put totally asleep or have a regional anesthetic which numbs just the leg involved. The latter is most popular, and it usually involves a supplemental agent administered intravenously which puts you into a light sleep. Within hours of the surgery, all the effects of the anesthesia are gone and you can walk out of the hospital fairly alert.

However, you will need someone to meet you at the hospital to bring you home.

Immediately prior to the operation, your surgeon will use your legs as a blackboard. As you stand on your feet, he will use a pen to mark exactly where each varicosity is located. These markings are needed because during the operation, the foot of the operating table is tilted up to empty the veins and the varicosities disappear. Emptying the leg veins with a tilted operating table also minimizes blood loss and makes it extremely unlikely you will need a transfusion. In fact, transfusions are exceedingly rare because the blood loss in this kind of surgery is minimal.

The first incision is made on the bikini line in the groin. It will be two to three inches long and fairly shallow because it need only reach the vein. Another incision of one-half to a full inch is made on the inner side of the leg near the ankle. Other incisions are made over each varicosity along the leg, each a half an inch or less.

The vascular surgeon will make three to four incisions in each leg. Until the mid-1980s, surgeons made dozens of tiny incisions over every visible varicosity, but they have come to realize that this number of cuts is unnecessary in most cases because after the defective saphenous vein is removed, most residual varicosities disappear within several months. (As already noted, any remaining varicosities can be dealt with effectively by injection therapy in your surgeon's office or a clinic.)

After the incisions are made, the doctor will insert an instrument known as a "vein stripper" into the saphenous vein, which starts at the ankle and ends in the groin. He passes the stripper all the way through to the other end and then pulls it back. As he tugs on the instrument, the vein comes with it. (This action is similar to putting your hand into a sock, expanding your fingers and then turning the sock inside out.) Your doctor then closes all incisions. As the stripper moves through your vein, your doctor will tie off the perforator veins that link the saphenous with the deep veins. By removing the saphenous veins, the doctor permanently interrupts the flow of blood through the perforators, forcing the blood to travel through the deep veins that already carry almost 90% of your venous blood back to the heart.

Does all this cutting leave scars? Not necessarily. Some scars disappear completely; others remain as fine, almost invisible, lines.

In the hands of a good vascular surgeon, these tiny superficial cuts virtually disappear when they heal. The end result is no more traumatic than wearing shorts and walking through prickly underbrush in the forest; your legs will get scratched up a bit, but they also will heal fast.

The final step in this process, which can take a total of one to three hours depending on whether one or both legs are done, is the bandaging. Your leg is wrapped in a sterile gauze dressing and an elastic Ace bandage is applied from the toes to the groin.

After the operation, you may stay in bed for several hours with your legs elevated on several pillows. However, by evening you will be home and you should walk five to ten minutes every hour until bedtime. Walking works the muscles that pump the veins and helps blood find new paths to the heart.

When you go home that evening, most surgeons will tell you to do whatever you wish, as long as it does not involve prolonged standing or sitting. Walking 5 to 10 minutes each hour is encouraged: the more walking, the better. In my practice, the leg remains bandaged for one week. I remove it at my patient's first post-operative office visit. Do not take the bandages off yourself; leave them on until your doctor removes them. Once the initial bandages are off, no more should be necessary. A simple Ace bandage, an elastic stocking or support hose should be worn if you are planning a long trip by car or plane within the first three months after your operation. You should wear the bandage or support hose only while you are traveling.

Post-operative pain should be minimal. Many patients describe a slight burning sensation around the incisions. Elevating your legs and taking a mild analgesic other than aspirin can help—the same cure used for puffy toes or ankles.

Elevating your legs once or twice a day should be part of your routine for the next few weeks after surgery. It aids healing and improves the appearance of the scars. Sometimes the operation can cause a black and blue discoloration (a blood spill under the skin). This discoloration is like a bruise and it will disappear within three to six weeks.

Overall, the recuperation period does not take as long as it once did. Patients get better faster now because doctors encourage them to start walking sooner. You should feel totally recuperated within two to three weeks and should be able to go back to work within two to three days, providing you take it easy and don't stand or sit too long.

Before we leave this section on surgery, let me add one note: Some of the latest innovations in vascular surgery are operations to repair the vein valves. One that some colleagues and I are doing involves banding the vein, or wrapping plastic around the exterior of the saphenous or deep vein where a valve is malfunctioning, and restoring the vein at this point to its normal diameter. This procedure forces the valve doors to close the way they should and prevents blood from flowing back down into the veins below. When these banding operations are done, some varicosities left in the veins need to be treated with sclerotherapy. Others need tiny cuts over the varicosed vein so a small part can be removed. So far, these operations are proving to be wonderful alternatives to the more extensive stripping surgery, but vascular surgeons need more of a track record with them to recommend the surgery on a wider scale.

We mentioned earlier that surgery is frequently performed to prevent the complications that come with varicose veins. Now it's time to explore those complications.

Notes

There is a lot of literature available that discusses which treatments are most appropriate under varying circumstances. Three articles to consult are "Symposium: Management of Varicose Veins" in *Contemporary Surgery* (June 1975); "Varicose Veins" by R. May in a 1985 book *Surgery of the Veins*, published by Grune & Stratton; and "Help for the patient with problem veins" by Howard C. Baron, Victor deWolfe, John A. Spittell and Edwin Wylie in *Patient Care* (March 1974).

Two interesting articles on elastic stockings—how modern ones were developed by an engineer, Conrad Jobst, for his own varicose veins and how the legs react to different stockings depending on how they are woven—are in *Surgery of the Veins* (cited above). They were written by John J. Bergan and George Johnson, respectively.

W.G. Fegan and John T. Hobbs have both written extensively on sclerotherapy and the use of compression therapy. For Fegan, a big fan of sclerotherapy, see "Continuous compression technique for injecting varicose veins" in *The Lancet* (1963); and *Varicose Veins: Compression Sclerotherapy*, a book published by Heinemann Medical Books in London in 1967. For Hobbs, see "Surgery and Sclerotherapy in the Treatment of Varicose Veins" in *Archives of Surgery* (December 1974) where he states that sclerotherapy is better for the superficial and perforator veins while surgery is preferable in the saphenous veins.

In addition to stripping and banding, vascular surgeons have experimented for the last 20 years with vein valve transplants and repairs. They also have tried transplanting or substituting whole veins and portions of them. For a discussion of their relative merits, see "Vein valve transplant for venous stasis disease" by David Calcagno and Peter Gloviczki in *Contemporary Surgery* (March 1989); "Valvuloplasty and valve transfer" by Seshadri Raju in *International Angiology* (1985); and "Long-term results of venous valve reconstruction: A four to twenty-one-year follow up" by Elna Masuda and Robert Kistner in *Journal of Vascular Surgery* (March 1994).

For more on sclerotherapy, the best book is Mitchel Goldman's *Sclerotherapy Treatment of Varicose and Telangiectatic Leg Veins* (published 1991 by Mosby–Year Book, Inc.).

CHAPTER 6

■■■■■■■■■■■■■■■■■■■■■■■■■■■■■■■■

COMPLICATIONS WITH
VARICOSE VEINS

A week before Christmas, Rose W., 74, became alarmed when her left ankle started bleeding profusely. By the time an ambulance arrived, she had saturated several towels. She wound up spending two days in the hospital before she was stable enough to return home where she lived alone. Her bleeding was caused by a ruptured varicose vein near the site of an operation that had been performed several days earlier to remove cancerous skin cells.

Rose's bleeding was an unusual complication from varicose veins, but it also had something in common with the more traditional complications: the ability to frighten you, disrupt your life, cost you money, and ultimately to kill you.

If Rose or her neighbor had not had the presence of mind to call an ambulance, Rose could have bled to death. Each year, a small but steady number of people (mostly elderly) die this way. Emergency rooms in New York City hospitals see at least one elderly patient a month bleeding from varicose veins.

Varicose veins are not a nuisance disease. They are a serious social and economic problem. Insidious in onset, their complications often require prolonged and extensive treatment. It is estimated that more than two million working days are lost in the U.S. because of chronic venous insufficiency and many of those are complications associated with varicose veins. About 10% of those who suffer from chronic venous insufficiency wind up in a hospital for treatment of some complication.

If you have varicose veins, this chapter may scare you or confuse you. It should do neither if you keep two things in mind:

1. Many of the symptoms for the complications associated with varicose veins are similar. Don't try to diagnose yourself; leave that to your doctor.

2. Don't delay in getting help, because one complication will often lead to another and another, setting off a chain reaction.

These complications can develop within days of each other and each new one can be more dangerous than the last.

The most common route of succession is: varicosities—phlebitis—thrombophlebitis—deep vein thrombosis—permanent leg swelling—a leg ulcer—migrating thrombosis—pulmonary embolus. Now, before your eyes glaze, remember your Greek, from which a lot of medical terminology is derived. *Phlebo* means vein; *thrombo* means clot; *-osis* means condition or process; and any word with *-itis* added to the end means inflammation or infection of the anatomical structure it describes. Thus, phlebitis means an inflamed vein; thrombophlebitis is an inflamed vein with a thrombus or clot in it; deep vein thrombosis refers to a clot in the deep leg veins; and, migrating thrombosis means that the clot or thrombus is traveling through the venous system. In the venous system, the last stop is the lungs and a pulmonary embolus is a clot that strikes there. Most people with varicose veins do not wind up with potentially dangerous clots in their lungs. Nevertheless, each year more than 150,000 people die in the U.S. from a pulmonary embolism, most within the first hour after the clot strikes the lungs.

The most common complications of varicose veins are phlebitis or thrombophlebitis, hemorrhage, varicose pigmentation and venous or stasis ulceration. Pulmonary embolisms, deep vein thrombosis and the post-thrombotic syndrome are problems, too, but they are seen less frequently. It is important to remember that each patient is an individual and complications in one can have different origins than complications in another. What follows is a description of the most common complications and their treatment. Each complication is treated as a separate condition even though all complications are related. The common denominator, of course, is the underlying problem—varicose veins.

Phlebitis

One of the most common complications of varicose veins, phlebitis is an inflamed vein wall. Generally, everybody who has varicose veins has an attack of phlebitis in one or more of their varicosities. Phlebitis usually occurs in one of the superficial veins: the branches of the greater saphenous vein that run up the inside of your calf and thigh, or the lesser saphenous vein, which starts on the outside of your ankles and moves up the back of your calf to the knee.

The first sign of phlebitis is often a dull ache, sometimes accompanied by a slight swelling of the lower leg or ankle and an area of tenderness along the course of the vein involved. The next stage affects the skin over the vein, which becomes pink and is warm and tender. With acute phlebitis, the skin is red and hot to the touch, and the limb hurts when squeezed or pressed.

In general, anyone with varicose veins should be aware of the symptoms of phlebitis. The onset is apt to be sudden, painful and debilitating. The pain can be mild and localized over the vein, or it can be so severe that it affects an entire portion of the leg. It can also cause weakness, fever, chills and a loss of appetite when the phlebitis worsens and becomes thrombophlebitis.

The treatment for localized phlebitis is generally conservative. Doctors will tell you to walk and/or go about your daily business wearing elastic support stockings. For at least one hour each day, you will be told to rest with your legs elevated above your heart so the veins can drain. You will be advised against prolonged sitting or standing.

Aspirin is usually prescribed for patients who are not allergic to it because it helps to prevent clots that can lead to more serious complications. Often, an anti-inflammatory drug will be prescribed. As the inflammation subsides, the redness in the skin over the affected vein gradually recedes and becomes tan or brown. The brown patch may disappear eventually, or it could become a permanent discoloration.

The worst way of treating phlebitis is putting the patient to bed, immobilized and given an inadequate dose of an anticoagulant. The treatment for phlebitis is to keep the patient active; immobilization is wrong and can result in the further spread of phlebitis from the superficial saphenous system into the deep veins. Keeping a phlebitic patient immobile can turn what should be a short benign illness into a protracted, serious illness with long-term consequences.

Phlebitis is most likely to occur if you have large, tortuous varicose veins and one of the following conditions: injury to the affected leg; pregnancy; an insect bite on the leg; athlete's foot; a previous bout with a thrombotic condition; prolonged bed rest for a chronic disease; obesity; and pooling of blood in the leg because of prolonged sitting. I've had patients develop phlebitis after returning from wonderful vacations that took them half way around the world; the long plane ride back where they spent hours sitting in confined positions caused their blood to pool and their veins to become inflamed.

Phlebitis is not usually a big problem when it occurs alone. Doctors get concerned with it when it develops into thrombophlebitis.

Thrombophlebitis

When a thrombus forms in an inflamed saphenous vein, the condition is called thrombophlebitis. It is a common complication of varicose veins. To understand thrombophlebitis, you have to know a little about blood chemistry. Your bloodstream has about 2.5 billion platelets—small, colorless, disklike cells. Normally, they speed through your veins without sticking to the interior walls because both the platelets and vein walls have a negative electrical charge and only opposite electrical charges attract. However, when the inner lining of your vein is damaged or injured or irregularly shaped because of a varicosity or for some other reason, the wall loses some of its negative charge and some platelets can stick to the site of the injury or irregularity. As the platelets pile on top of each other, they form a thrombus, a tough, gray, semitransparent mass that sticks to the wall of a blood vessel.

A thrombus is not a blood clot. It is more solid and tougher than a clot and it only forms in a vein where the blood continues to flow; a clot develops in static, pooled blood. However, a thrombus can help to create a clot by slowing the flow of blood and causing it to pool in the vicinity of the site of the thrombus.

The symptoms of thrombophlebitis are a lot like those of phlebitis. You feel a dull ache, sometimes with a slight swelling of your calf or ankle. Your skin can be itchy and warm and tender to touch and it hurts when the affected area of your leg is pressed or squeezed. You can feel a hard, cord-like swelling along the affected vein. You also can experience weakness, fever, chills and a loss of appetite.

The public generally doesn't hear much about thrombophlebitis until it strikes a well-known figure, like the late President Richard

Nixon. However, thrombophlebitis is far more common than is generally recognized. Like phlebitis, it can be triggered by surgery, insect bites, pregnancy, etc. Dr. John Spittell, a consultant in cardiovascular disease at the Mayo Clinic in Rochester, Minnesota, estimates that up to 40% of all people who have any kind of surgery develop thrombophlebitis. It has been my experience that the presence of varicose veins before surgery makes it far more likely that thrombophlebitis will develop.

Doctors disagree about the extent to which thrombophlebitis is dangerous. Some say it's not. They argue that the clots do not travel when they start in the saphenous veins. Harold Dodd and Frank Cockett, two renowned English vascular surgeons who wrote a definitive book on diseases that affect veins in the lower limbs, disagree:

> "Superficial thrombosis in varicose veins has traditionally been regarded as a benign process without risk of pulmonary embolism. Nothing can be further from the truth! . . . A significant number of cases of pulmonary embolism (potentially fatal blood clots in the lung) originate in the first instance in an attack of superficial thrombophlebitis which has spread into the deep veins."

The professionals' disagreement about the dangers of thrombophlebitis also extends to how it should be treated. Doctors who feel it is not dangerous recommend hot packs, aspirin, possibly an anticoagulating drug and support hose. However, Dodd and Cockett advise doctors to treat thrombophlebitis like an emergency and operate "within a day or so of onset." They recommend a localized thrombectomy that removes that area of the vein that contains the thrombophlebitis. If surgery has to be delayed, you should be advised to have an elective thrombectomy as soon as possible.

I believe that the treatment depends on the severity of the condition and the general health of the patient. For some, if surgery is not immediately possible, a more conservative approach to treatment—wrapping the leg in an Ace bandage or fitted elastic stocking, getting the patient to walk and take aspirin—may be appropriate. However, for others this approach means playing with a time bomb. Surgery would be absolutely necessary at the first sign that a thrombus is moving upward.

Whatever the treatment, thrombophlebitis should not be ignored, or it will spread and become a long-term serious problem.

Deep Vein Thrombosis

When a thrombus or clot forms deep in the veins, you have a serious problem called deep vein thrombosis. There are many reasons why deep vein thrombosis develops and some have nothing to do with varicose veins. This condition can be caused by a trauma, malignancy or infection. You can be genetically predisposed to getting these clots and have the condition triggered by obesity or a sedentary lifestyle. A less common cause is polycythaemia, a disease that causes your bone marrow to produce too many red blood cells. Most typically, it occurs in a hospitalized patient as a complication from some illness that requires a long bed rest. Perhaps the most common cause is surgery, especially in geriatric patients in the post-op period following hip or knee reconstruction. It is estimated that 40%–70% of these patients develop deep vein thrombosis and for 25% of these patients, the first sign that they have this potentially deadly complication is when they develop a pulmonary embolism.

Varicose veins also can cause deep vein thrombosis. If you have varicose veins, you can get deep vein thrombosis from a case of thrombophlebitis in the saphenous veins. In this instance, a thrombus or clot moves from a saphenous vein through a perforator vein into one of your deep veins.

Nobody knows for sure how often varicose veins result in deep vein thrombosis. Whether varicose veins are the direct cause or not, certain factors associated with varicose veins are always found with deep vein thrombosis. These include blood pooling, injury to the inner lining of a vein and an increased clotting tendency.

Doctors do agree, though, that vein thrombosis is a potentially serious complication because your deep leg veins are on a straight path to your heart and lungs. They also agree that deep vein thrombosis is difficult to detect because simple tests like an X ray are not definitive and, as mentioned above, often the first sign of a deep vein thrombosis comes after the clot has moved and damaged your heart or lungs. Dr. Lazar Greenfield, professor and chairman of surgery at the University of Michigan Hospitals in Ann Arbor, estimates that there is no warning of a deep vein

thrombosis about 60% of the time. (See the next section on pulmonary embolism.) When you do get any kind of advance warning, the
symptoms can be misleading. You might have the symptoms of
thrombophlebitis—tenderness, swelling, warm skin over a limited
area of your leg—or a low grade fever.

Deep vein thrombosis most often occurs in the veins located in
the soleus muscle of your calf. The most important warning signs to
occur there are the sudden onset of swelling (often at the ankle) and
tenderness when the calf is squeezed. When an attack involves the
pelvic veins, the left leg is involved twice as often as the right and the
pain, swelling and tenderness often involves the entire leg.

Your doctor can confirm that you have deep vein thrombosis with
a doppler probe or venography. A radioactive fibrinogen test can
also confirm this; iodine is used to block your thyroid gland and
then blood samples are taken from different parts of your leg. High
levels of fibrinogen, as measured by this test, indicate that a
thrombus is growing in your veins because the radioactive material
is picked up by the clot. There also is a fairly reliable mechanical
test, called impedance plethysmography, that works like a blood
pressure device: a cuff is put around your thigh and inflated to
squeeze it. As the cuff is loosened, your doctor measures the blood
flow. If your blood doesn't flow fast enough, it is assumed that there
is a thrombus blocking the path.

The treatment for deep vein thrombosis can be medical or surgical.
The goal is the same: to prevent the thrombus from migrating to the
lung and to stop the clot from growing in the involved vein. Patients
often will be told first to rest in bed with their legs elevated to allow
the thrombus to attach itself more firmly to the vein wall. They will
be given Heparin, a blood thinner, intravenously. That might be
followed by oral doses of Coumarin, another kind of anticoagulant,
to prevent the formation of new clots. However, these drugs are not
for everyone.

If patients cannot take an anticoagulant drug or it doesn't work
well enough to prevent new clots or a thrombus from migrating to
the lung, then surgery is in order. Surgery could involve a thrombectomy, the removal of the clot or thrombus from your vein. This
procedure is generally used to minimize limb swelling and prevent
further growth of the clot or thrombus. Doctors prefer to do a

thrombectomy when the clot is less than two to three days old. Often this approach is not feasible due to a lack of symptoms.

After you have had a clot for more than several days, thrombectomies are not possible. At this point, it is far more likely that your vascular surgeon will want to install a device designed to impede the flow of a clot through your vena cava, the main vein bringing blood from your lower extremities to your heart. This is something like putting a screen over your kitchen drain to prevent scraps of food from getting into your pipes. Some of these devices are placed around the outside of the vena cava. More popular intraluminal gadgets are inserted into the vena cava (usually through the jugular vein in the neck). For years, one intraluminal caval filter, designed by Lazar Greenfield, has had the approval of the U.S. Food and Drug Administration, but others are being tested and are on their way to being permitted by the FDA. When in place and open, the Greenfield filter looks like a tiny umbrella that has been denuded and twisted in a wind storm.

Two final points should be made about deep vein thrombosis: When it occurs, symptoms might show up in only one leg while a deadly clot is moving quietly up the other. In addition, deep vein thrombosis permanently damages the valves in your leg veins and usually leads within five years to a variety of problems, such as persistent aching and swelling and repeated ankle ulcers. Post-thrombotic syndrome will be discussed later in this chapter.

Pulmonary Embolism

One minute you seem healthy. The next minute you have chest pain, a cough, shortness of breath, tachypnea (rapid, often shallow breathing) and great anxiety. A heart attack? Maybe. But it also could be a pulmonary embolism.

A pulmonary embolism occurs when a clot breaks loose from a vein wall and travels through the right side of your heart through the pulmonary artery to your lung. When it gets stuck in your lung, it reduces the amount of freshly oxygenated blood returning to the left side of your heart. Depending on the size of the clot and other factors, a pulmonary embolism can kill you.

The American Medical Association estimates that there are 650,000 cases of pulmonary embolism in the U.S. each year and about 30% of those result in death. It is estimated that 90% of those emboli get their start in the lower extremities and more than half of those start in the legs, often the calf veins.

The causes are a lot like those mentioned above for deep vein thrombosis, including trauma, tumors and surgery. Some researchers say five of every 1,000 adults undergoing major surgery will die from a massive pulmonary embolism. Rudolf Virchow, the great German pathologist of the 19th century, was the first to explain why pulmonary emboli originate in the lower extremities. In what became known as Virchow's triad, he said three conditions are needed for a thrombus to form: damage to a vein wall or lining, slowing or pooling of blood in a vein and a change in the coagulability or clotting of blood. People with varicose veins have all the conditions of Virchow's triad: a damaged, distended vein in which a malfunctioning valve allows blood to pool and ultimately clot.

You can suffer from pulmonary embolism without having any sign of varicose veins, but the presence of varicosities, or a history of them, greatly increases the risk and makes it more likely that the attack will be fatal. Many people have no warning of a pulmonary embolism. About half of those who die from pulmonary embolism had no warning at all. Others have nonfatal attacks that are seen as a warning that more can come. About 30% of those who have nonfatal attacks will experience another pulmonary embolism. Still others experience a pulmonary embolism but never even know it because the clots are so small that they don't produce the kind of dramatic symptoms described above—chest pain, breathlessness, etc.—or other symptoms, such as coughing up blood. (All these come after an embolism has already hit its mark.)

When patients do have these symptoms, doctors can have difficulty diagnosing a pulmonary embolism because the symptoms are very similar to those of heart and other chest disorders. One of the most reliable signs of migrating emboli is a sudden rise in the pulse rate, often accompanied by a drop in blood pressure and the patient's feeling faint. Because of the overall uncertainty of the situation, doctors will want to do many tests: Xrays (to look for wedge-shaped scarring in the lungs); an electrocardiogram (to measure heartbeats); a pulmonary angiogram (in which blood vessels running through the lungs are injected with dye and X-rayed to show signs of blockages); and blood gas measurements. If your doctor suspects the cause is deep vein thrombosis of the legs, he may do a Doppler study and a venogram of both legs to pinpoint the site and size of the thrombus.

The goal of any treatment is to prevent the thrombus from growing and additional emboli from forming.

At first, your doctor will order you to have complete bed rest in a hospital with your legs elevated. He also will prescribe anticlotting drugs such as Heparin, which must be taken intravenously, and then Coumarin, which can be taken orally. The bed rest regimen might last as much as a week with the goal of allowing the thrombus to attach itself more firmly to the vein wall. For the next few months, the doctor may prescribe elastic support hose.

Heparin, Coumarin and other anticoagulating drugs prevent new clots from forming, but they don't dissolve old ones. A new group of drugs called thrombolytic agents can dissolve clots as well. Your doctor might prescribe one of those alone or in combination with an anticoagulant. Another kind of drug your doctor might prescribe is one that prevents blood platelets from forming a thrombus. (Remember: a thrombus and blood clot are not the same thing.) Of this group of drugs, aspirin is the most frequently used, especially when long-term treatment is necessary.

Surgery to remove the clot from a lung is rare, but doctors are increasingly resorting to the installation of a filter in the vena cava to interrupt the upward movement of the thrombi. Vena caval interruption and thrombectomy are the alternatives when bed rest and drugs don't work. Surgery also is in order if the thrombus is in the thigh or higher and poses an imminent danger.

Milk Leg and Blue Leg

Before discussing the long-term complications that can result from a thrombus or clot in your leg veins, it's worth spending a little time on two potentially dangerous conditions that are offshoots of deep-vein thrombosis: milk leg (phlegmasia alba dolens) and blue leg (phlegmasia caerulea dolens).

Milk leg is another form of deep vein thrombosis. It is called milk leg when it occurs in a woman who has just given birth. (The name stems from the mistaken belief that milk produced by nursing mothers eventually settled in their legs.) Like deep vein thrombosis, it is the result of a phlebitis attack in the femoral vein (the deep vein in the thigh) and the popliteal vein (in the lower leg).

The symptoms of milk leg are that your leg suddenly turns white, swells and hurts. When the thrombus and inflammation are in your femoral vein, your leg—starting in the thigh—will feel tense and hot. If a thrombus is in your popliteal vein, your calf and foot will be tender and swollen. One good thing about milk leg: The symptoms are vivid and demand immediate attention. They can include pain toward the back of the knee and calf, plus tense, shiny, pale skin.

Treatment involves elevating the leg, applying heat, anticoagulant drugs and sometimes anti-inflammatory drugs. If you have to be active, your lower limb should be encased in an elastic bandage or stocking. Often an elastic leotard is ideal because it compresses the leg veins and supports the lower abdomen as well. If this conservative approach doesn't work, your doctor could recommend a thrombectomy, the surgical removal of clots from the affected veins. Surgery minimizes the danger of pulmonary embolism and reduces the possibility of chronic or permanent damage to veins in the lower limb.

The symptoms and consequences of blue leg are more alarming than they are for white leg. With blue leg, your entire leg can become swollen, painful, warm and pale blue within a few hours.

If you try to ignore these warnings, the circulation in your foot will slow and could shut down completely. Gradually, your foot and the lower part of your leg become badly swollen and cold, the blue color intensifies. Eventually, dark, sinister-looking blisters can erupt on your toes and foot and gangrene can infect your lower leg. One possible consequence of gangrene is the amputation of the affected limb.

Fortunately, only 10% of those who have deep vein thrombosis ever experience serious complications like these.

Post-Thrombotic Syndrome

If you have deep vein thrombosis, particularly in the illiofemoral vein (where the thigh meets the groin), it's likely that you will experience post-thrombotic syndrome. It is a variety of problems that occur simultaneously. They include swelling (edema), hardening, pain and ulcers, all in the lower leg. Another condition is dermatitis, in which the skin around the lower leg itches, weeps and appears irritated.

These problems can be mild or severe, but they all develop within five years of deep vein thrombosis if the patient does not go to a doctor until after the latent period has elapsed.

Dodd and Cockett (the doctors who wrote the definitive textbook on diseases of the lower limb veins *(The Pathology and Surgery of the Lower Limb)*, estimate that "up to 75% of people who have had thrombosis of the deep veins of the legs suffer for the rest of their lives" from this syndrome.

The syndrome develops because deep vein thrombosis causes permanent damage to the vein valves in your lower leg, particularly in the perforator veins that connect the saphenous and deep veins. The malfunctioning valves allow venous blood to pool in your lower limbs, causing pressure to build in the small veins of your lower leg, ankle and foot. As this pressure builds, fluid seeps from the smaller vessels and capillaries, drowning layers of tissue under the skin.

Swelling around the ankle is the first sign of post-thrombotic syndrome. Initially, the swelling will disappear after a night's rest. Gradually, however, the swelling does not go away and the soft tissue and fat layers normally situated under the skin are replaced by tough, fibrous tissue that is hard compared to healthy tissue.

You can tell an ulcer is about to erupt when your ankle and the inner or outer sides of your leg are persistently red. The ulcer can be triggered by minor injuries like cuts, insect bites or bumps. These can cause a break in skin that is essentially being deprived of a normal, healthy blood flow. When the wound refuses to heal, it can gradually become an ulcer that also is very difficult to heal. According to one study, 300,000 to 400,000 Americans have venous ulcers (about 1% of the population) and most of them are women.

Treatment usually consists of wearing elastic bandages or support stockings, which help prevent blood from pooling in veins that feed skin tissue. In addition, your doctor might order a daily period of leg elevation (to drain the veins) and no prolonged periods of standing or sitting. These measures combined with exercise often are enough to provide a long term cure—providing the syndrome is detected in its early stages before an ulcer erupts. However, once you have an ulcer, treatment becomes more complicated.

Rolled bandages and different kinds of plasters were prescribed for leg ulcers since before the birth of Christ. Roman doctors also were known to have anointed leg ulcers with antiseptic healing wines.

In 1815, J. Hodgson, an English doctor, firmly established the link that Hippocrates, the father of medicine, had noticed 2,000 years ago: that leg ulcers develop in legs with varicose veins.

Doctors will initially try to treat a leg ulcer with the conservative measures described above: leg elevation and elastic bandages. Another method, developed toward the end of the 19th century by a German dermatologist, Paul Gerson Unna, is the Unna paste boot. Lighter and more flexible than the standard plaster cast, the Unna boot is made of zinc oxide and glycerin applied to a roll-on bandage. The Unna boot keeps the leg slightly immobilized, leg varicosities compressed and the ulcer crater medicated. Finally, it keeps your hands away from the ulcer, making it easier for you to resist poking, scratching or applying some home remedy that could make the situation worse.

Even after your ulcer is cured (and it can be a time consuming process), you may need surgery to prevent it from erupting again. One operation involves putting a skin graft over the ulcer. A second operation could be performed to remove the veins with the malfunctioning valves.

There are an estimated 2.5 million Americans suffering from chronic venous insufficiency, and 300,000 to 400,000 of these get these troubling ulcers.

Hemorrhage

This chapter opened with a description of Rose W.'s startling discovery that her left ankle was bleeding profusely. Rose's frightening condition was a hemorrhage, a situation where blood gushes from an injured vessel. Hemorrhages used to be relatively rare. In recent years, though, spontaneous hemorrhages from varicose veins have become more common because we are living longer and the circulatory system evolved for a shorter life span.

If you have varicose veins and suddenly discover your foot or shoe is wet with blood, lie flat and elevate your leg immediately. Have someone apply a pressure dressing directly over the site and then call a doctor. Do NOT try to block the flow of blood above the wound by applying a tourniquet. This technique could actually increase the bleeding because your venous blood, flowing upward back to your heart, would have nowhere to flow except out of the body.

A tourniquet above the wound could damage leg tissues, especially in older people, by compressing arterial flow.

Now that the complications of the disease have been explored, the next chapter explains why women have more problems with their veins than men.

Notes

Complications are not the norm with varicose veins as long as the condition is not neglected. Unfortunately, too many do neglect them, out of ignorance, lack of insurance coverage, misdiagnosis, or for other reasons.

The frequencies cited in this chapter are culled from a variety of sources. For example, the estimate of workdays lost to chronic deep venous insufficiency and the percent of people who need to be hospitalized for this problem are cited in a paper "Chronic Deep Venous Insufficiency" by Kenneth J. Cherry and Larry H. Hollier. The estimates of how many people die from pulmonary embolism come from the American Medical Association's *Family Medical Guide* and Lazar Greenfield, a doctor who designed a well regarded trap that is installed in the vena cava to prevent a clot from a leg vein moving up to the lung. Both peg the number of deaths caused by pulmonary embolism to approximately 200,000 per year in the U.S. The estimate that up to 400,000 Americans have venous leg ulcers comes from an article by Thomas F. O'Donnell Jr. in "Chronic Venous Insufficiency and Varicose Veins."

In the context of this book, what's important here is these complications can be deadly and a lot of people, capable doctors included, often don't draw the connection between the symptoms and complications that come from varicose veins and other life-threatening problems.

For example, Greenfield and Barbara Michna, in a chapter they wrote in *Surgery of the Veins*, report that pulmonary embolism is **misdiagnosed as much as 70% of the time**; 90% to 95% of the emboli come from the lower extremities, and half of these come from below the inguinal ligament.

They also point out that 30% of the patients who don't realize they've had a pulmonary embolism and don't get treatment will have another attack.

Most of the Greenfield-Michna chapter is devoted to the relative merits of several mechanical devices used to catch clots as they travel from the legs toward the lungs.

Meanwhile, the *Journal of Cardiovascular Surgery*, in 1988, ran an article by Thomas Nash, who concluded that vein valve transplants were a good long-term solution for leg ulcers, which tend to occur in people with malfunctioning popliteal vein valves. He also said it was a good solution for those with pre-ulcer skin problems.

CHAPTER 7

■■■■■■■■■■■■■■■■■■■■■■■■■■■■■■■■■■

WOMEN ESPECIALLY

Women are far more apt to get varicose veins than men. Some doctors estimate that varicosities strike women four to one over men. Others think it's two to one. Whatever the difference, women seem to be particularly vulnerable to varicose veins at two critical physiological milestones in their lives: pregnancy and menopause.

This timing makes doctors believe that female sex hormones play a role in triggering varicose veins. Some researchers believe that excess estrogen can spark varicose veins; others think the level of progesterone is key. Hormonal levels surge and recede dramatically during pregnancy and menopause.

This chapter takes a look at what is known or suspected about the relationships between varicose veins and both pregnancy and menopause, and how hormones affect the veins of women. First, we will take a quick look at some of the myths and realities about varicose veins and pregnancy. After that, we offer a brief explanation of what these female sex hormones are, how they work in healthy women and more specifically, how they affect their veins. Then, we will tackle the issue of how hormones in birth control pills work and whether they are advisable for women with varicose veins. Finally, we will deal with pregnant and menopausal women who have varicosities, how to treat pregnant women with varicose veins and whether hormone replacement therapy is safe for menopausal women with varicose veins.

One of the most vivid examples in medical history of pregnancy-related varicose veins involves Queen Anne of England, who reigned from 1702 to 1714. Her saga is a classic case of wealth without health. Pregnant 17 times in 16 years, she lost every child, most within a few days of their birth, some before term. The one who survived infancy was horribly deformed and hidden until he died, probably from a plague, shortly after his twelfth birthday. Fat and in severe pain most of the time, Anne was in such poor health that she had to be carried to the throne for her coronation at age 37. She subsequently held many Sunday morning cabinet meetings from her bed.

Queen Anne's doctors attributed her pain to gout or ague (probably a reference to malaria) and they fought over who was responsible. However, judging from the symptoms, we are now virtually certain that Anne suffered from varicose veins and developed severe complications because of her weight and multiple pregnancies. Before she died at 49, her doctors' records report that her face was constantly red and spotted and her affected foot "tied up with poultice and some hasty bandages." Her left leg, inflamed from foot to ankle, had a varicose ulcer. The cause of her death is believed to be a blood clot in her lung, a complication of her varicosed legs.

Don't assume from this anecdote that pregnancy caused Queen Anne's varicose veins. Pregnancy does not cause varicose veins. However, it can trigger them in women who are predisposed to having them.

Pregnancy brings on varicose veins in several ways. One is the weight of a growing fetus in the womb. As the uterus expands, it can start to impede the flow of blood through the abdomen and, in effect, force it back into the leg veins. The expanding volume of blood in pregnant women also puts more pressure on the leg veins, triggering the eruption of dormant varicosities. However, very often the first signals women have that they are pregnant are the symptoms of varicose veins: aching, tired, weak legs, possibly swollen and with spider veins or blue knots erupting. Those signs often turn up in the first weeks of pregnancy, well before the uterus grows heavy or the mother's supply of blood increases. These early signs prompted scientists to start looking for other reasons for pregnancy-related varicose veins and why they have come to settle on hormones.

Hormones

Hormones are chemicals made by organs known as endocrine glands. Everyone has four basic glands: the pituitary (in the brain); the thyroid and parathyroid (in the neck); the adrenal (on top of the kidneys); and the pancreas (which lays over one kidney). In addition, women get hormones from their ovaries and men from their testes. Hormones from these glands go directly into the bloodstream and work with the nervous system to help insure that various organs and tissues throughout the body function as one big coordinated machine.

Your body's hormonal levels change in response to different needs and events, such as the onset of a high fever or a pregnancy. Estrogen and progesterone are just two of many hormones produced by the endocrine glands, but they are the ones that most concern doctors who specialize in problems of the venous system.

Estrogen and progesterone are produced by the adrenal glands and by the ovaries; in healthy women, the level of these hormones rises and falls in tune with their bodies' cyclical changes. For example, when women are about to menstruate, their progesterone level rises. As they start bleeding, it subsides and estrogen rises, particularly at midcycle when their ovaries release eggs. Progesterone also soars in the first two weeks of a pregnancy. After that, estrogen escalates and stays at above normal levels until the pregnancy ends.

As women approach menopause, their estrogen and progesterone levels surge and recede at erratic intervals, causing headaches, hot flashes and a whole assortment of side effects. Doctors in Oxford, England, report that many signs of premenstrual syndrome intensify just before menopause arrives and women confuse this sharper form of PMS with the discomforts of menopause. PMS is believed to be directly linked to hormonal levels, but researchers disagree as to whether it is due to excesses or shortages of estrogen or progesterone.

Estrogen and progesterone appear to have an impact on the veins in a number of ways. One theory holds that estrogen or progesterone or both stretch the veins by changing the structure of the muscle in the vein walls. A.M. McCausland, a doctor at the University of Southern California School of Medicine, noted as early as 1963 that when these hormones are found at elevated levels in the blood, the veins expand. He and his colleagues found that during the menstrual cycle, there is a 20%–30% increase in "venous distensibility," and a 150% increase during pregnancy.

Another theory suggests that high levels of estrogen and progesterone in your blood affect your veins by changing the chemistry of your blood. In a 1992 paper for the International Journal of Fertility, Daniel Mishell, a professor of obstetrics and gynecology at the University of Southern California, said birth control pills, which contain various amounts of estrogen, are now known to cause "an increase in the hepatic production of serum globulins," some of which are "involved in coagulation." In other words, doctors think some oral contraceptives can cause clots to form in the blood of certain women.

Lila Nachtigall, a prominent endocrinologist in New York City, reports that oral contraceptives, which have high doses of estrogen, in effect decrease those chemicals in the blood that fight clots. This finding is now thought to explain why oral contraceptives seem to trigger venous thrombosis, strokes and/or heart attacks in some users.

So what is it? Do the hormones affect the muscle structure of the veins or do they change the chemistry of your blood? To evaluate these theories, it's worth looking at the development of oral contraceptives and seeing how women's bodies are affected when you tinker with their hormonal levels.

Oral Contraceptives

Since the beginning of medicine, doctors have looked for the ideal contraceptive—one that would be reliable, harmless, simple, practical, universally applicable and satisfactory both to men and women.

Hippocrates, the father of medicine, had one approach: "If a woman does not wish to become pregnant, dissolve in water misy as large as a bean and give it to her to drink, and for a year, she will not become pregnant." Unfortunately, he didn't leave a recipe for misy (an ancient Greek remedy), so no one today has any idea what he was talking about.

In ancient China, according to John Camp in his book *Magic, Myth and Medicine*, priestesses in the temples where sexual intercourse was part of the religious ceremony were reported to have taken white lead in large quantities for its contraceptive properties. (Do not try this. Lead poisoning is unpleasant and sometimes fatal.)

Norman Himes in his *Medical History of Contraception* says that St. Jerome Hieronymous, a father of the church, condemned (and thus confirmed the existence of) people in the fourth and fifth centuries who drank potions to bring on sterility.

In the last 200 years, it has been the business community (particularly the drug companies), not medical science, that has made the bigger strides in developing contraceptives. Ironically, the pill as we know it was created as an effort to *encourage* conception, not to avoid it—and in cows, not people! There are few things more frustrating to a farmer than a sterile cow, and so the story goes, the pill is an outgrowth of efforts by farmers in the early 1800s to reverse sterility in cows. According to Doctors Joseph Goldzieher and Harry Rudel, two Swiss scientists writing for the *Journal of the American Medical Association*, farmers understood that an ovarian abnormality was a major cause of infertility in cattle. They also understood that it could be reversed. By operating on the cows and manually crushing yellow cells around the animal's ovaries, the farmers found that they could often make the cows fertile again. The farmers, however, did not know why this procedure worked, but today we do. Crushing these yellow cells, or corpus luteum, destroyed the cow's source of progesterone so that the pituitary could resume telling the ovary to send out a new egg. The reason that this method worked was not figured out until the turn of the century when a French histologist, Prenant, at the University of Nancy, correctly theorized that the corpus luteum produced a hormone.

In 1927, Ludwig Haberlandt, professor of physiology at Innsbruck, Austria, discovered that if he took extracts from the ovary and fed it to mice, he could produce temporary sterility. Haberlandt correctly theorized that progesterone was nature's way of preventing a woman from getting pregnant again until she gives birth. In other words, **progesterone is nature's own secret birth control device.** Unfortunately, progesterone was difficult to obtain. Until the 1940s, it was selling for $200 a gram (or $440,000 a pound). Then Russell Marker, a chemist, went to Mexico's mountains and found a wild plant, cabezas de negro, that would let him produce progesterone cheaply. He returned to the U.S. with two large jars of progesterone worth between one-quarter and one-half a million dollars. However, Marker was a better researcher than businessman; several efforts that he made to produce and market oral contraceptives failed.

Since World War II, however, drug companies around the world have succeeded in marketing oral contraceptives. Since they were introduced on a large scale in the 1960s, birth control pills have been used by 150 million women worldwide (50 million in the U.S.). A 1988 study by one pharmaceutical firm found 13.8 million American women on the pill.

Today, most birth control pills prescribed in the U.S. contain both estrogen and progesterone. They are an outgrowth of research done in the 1950s by Gregory Pincus, an expert in hormonal research based at the Worcester Foundation for Experimental Biology in Shrewsbury, Massachusetts, who was invited by Planned Parenthood to find the ideal contraceptive.

Working with John Rock, a physician also based at the Worcester Foundation for Experimental Biology, Pincus found that progesterone alone was not enough. **Estrogen also acts as a natural contraceptive.** Pincus and Rock discovered that when the ovary releases an egg each month, it secretes estrogen which (like progesterone) also sends a signal to the pituitary to take a rest for a while.

Progesterone *and* estrogen, then, are nature's contraceptives and they remain in a woman's bloodstream for only a short time each month during the normal menstrual cycle. As soon as a woman becomes pregnant, they stay in her blood at elevated levels to protect her fertilized egg from potential competition from other eggs. In a sense, birth control pills work by fooling Mother Nature into thinking that a pregnancy already exists.

Side Effects

For some women, there are potentially serious side effects from taking the pill. They include increased risk of heart attack, stroke and thrombophlebitis. In 1967, the Royal College of General Practitioners showed in one of the first comprehensive studies on side effects of oral contraceptives that pill users had two to three times greater risk of thromboembolism than non-users. Subequent studies found that the risk was as much as 12 times greater for pill users.

Given this background, it's reasonable for those with varicose veins to wonder if they should take oral contraceptives. A particular worry is the fact that those who have varicose veins (like those who take the pill) have an increased chance of getting thrombophlebitis. Does taking the pill increase the chance of getting thrombophlebitis or other potentially dangerous complications for women with varicose veins?

In the past when my patients raised these issues, I told them that women with varicose veins, a history of phlebitis or a clotting disorder should not take oral contraceptives. Now, the answer is not so clear-cut because new birth control pills are safer than the old ones. Recent research shows that the risk of heart attacks and thrombophlebitis from oral contraceptives has dropped over the years as pharmaceutical companies have cut the amount of estrogen and progesterone used in their contraceptives.

Before 1973, most oral contraceptives had 50 mcg of ethinyl estradiol or 50–100 mcg of mestranol (two different kinds of estrogen). Today, most pills have 20–50 mcg of ethinyl estradiol. Meanwhile, the dose of progestogen in oral contraceptives dropped from 10 mg in 1960 to less than 1 mg by the late 1980s. In the last 15 years, according to Mishell in his 1992 paper, several studies have shown "the incidence of fatal or nonfatal embolic or thrombotic events was directly related to the estrogen dose." As the dose dropped, so did the number of heart attacks and strokes.

The reason is that, as noted before, elevated levels of estrogen in the bloodstream are now known to increase clotting factors. Less estrogen, fewer clots.

The challenge has been finding the right level of estrogen: Women need enough to prevent pregnancy but not so much that it causes clots to form. The pharmaceutical companies appear to have achieved the right balance in terms of avoiding heart attacks and strokes. The circumstances are not so clear when it comes to diseases of the venous system. It now looks like taking the pill itself will not necessarily increase your chance of venous thrombosis, but the picture is not so clear if you smoke or require surgery while on the pill.

In that 1992 study, Mishell cites one report that states the incidence of venous thrombosis is still three times greater for women using low estrogen contraceptives than for women using no oral contraceptives. Also, women who smoke and take low estrogen contraceptives have a still greater risk of venous thrombosis than non smokers. "Cigarette smoking acts synergistically with the estrogen-related hypercoagulability associated with arterial thrombosis, possibly due to the effect of nicotine on thromboxane release" in pill users,

Mishell writes. He cites one study which found that women currently taking the pill and smoking 15 or more cigarettes a day (less than a pack) were 20 times more likely to have a heart attack. Finally, Mishell reports, women who have major surgery or any illness or accidents that requires prolonged bed rest still have a much greater chance of experiencing a thromboembolism if they're taking the pill.

Mishell's findings would seem to support advice that doctors have given for years to women facing surgery or immobilization for any other reason: Stop taking oral contraceptives for at least one month before the operation.

Doctors who gave this advice also are getting reaffirmation from another 1992 report from Massachusetts General Hospital in Boston where researchers looked at more than 900 men and women suspected of having a pulmonary embolism. Doctors there found that women using oral contraceptives are not more likely to experience a pulmonary embolism. However, 80% of the pill users who underwent surgery subsequently developed an embolism compared with only 14% of the pill users who had no surgery and 12% of those who had surgery and were not taking the pill.

With studies like these in mind, I still think it is a good idea to err on the side of caution: If you are facing surgery or a period of immobilization for any reason (for example, you're trying to mend a broken ankle), stop taking the pill for a while. The break can't hurt (as long as you take other precautions to avoid pregnancy).

Now let's get back to the original question: Should women with varicose veins or a history of clotting or thrombophlebitis avoid oral contraceptives—even the new pills with less estrogen? Each case is different and needs to be evaluated by a doctor. One woman might have greater cause for concern than another because of her family's health history. Generally, I would say take the pill if the following conditions are present: your varicosities are not so serious that you're losing work or sleep from them; you are under 35; *and* you don't smoke. Otherwise, avoid it.

Pregnancy

Preventing pregnancy is one issue for women with varicose veins. Dealing with pregnancy and varicosities is another.

First, you should know that most of the symptoms of varicose veins that appear during pregnancy disappear within weeks of the birth. However, women who have varicose veins through multiple pregnancies have an increasingly difficult time getting their legs back to normal, and some never do so without surgery or sclerotherapy.

As noted before, there are three basic reasons why women get varicose veins when they are pregnant:

1) Increased levels of hormones, particularly estrogen, result in the relaxation of smooth muscles, enabling the uterus to expand to accommodate a baby. These hormones also soften the walls of the veins of pregnant women, making it tougher in some instances for those vein valves to close.

2) The veins are under much greater pressure because pregnant women have a much greater volume of blood flowing through their bodies. Blood volume increases more than four times in the first two months of pregnancy and doubles again in the third month.

3) Blood flow through veins in the abdomen can be impeded as the fetus and uterus grow, particularly during the third trimester when the fetus turns head down. The blood, then, backs up, putting greater pressure on the leg veins.

All these factors can result in visible varicosites that run from thigh to ankle; invisible and comparatively mild aching discomfort that goes away when the expectant mother puts her feet up; spider veins; or vulval varicosities on the labia, or vaginal lips, which look like a cluster of grapes and cause a lot of itching and burning.

It has been estimated that between 10% and 25% of all pregnant women get varicose veins. (However, it's likely that this number is rising as more and more women are waiting longer to have babies, and the older that women are—pregnant or not—the more vulnerable they are to varicose veins.) Burkitt, the English physician, offered one other observation in 1976 which puts this subject in perspective: Women in developing countries have far more pregnancies than women in the West, yet varicose veins are much more prevalent in the West. Just remember that virtually all the statistics in this book are based on women in the West.

There are three basic ways for pregnant women to deal with varicose veins: elastic, exercise and elevation, otherwise known as the three Es.

Elastic stockings help compress the leg veins, prevent them from dilating and keep those vein valves working properly so that blood cannot flow back down the legs and pool. Ordinary panty hose will not accomplish this task. Support hose is not recommended either, unless your problem is very minor. That's because support hose compresses your entire leg at one rate when the compression needs to be gradual—more at the ankle and less at the thigh. Special stockings fitted to your leg, and your expanding tummy, are best. They are expensive but worth the investment because taking care of varicose veins during pregnancy can help ensure a full recovery after your baby is born.

One more word on the stockings: They go on in the morning before you get out of bed and stay on until you retire for the night.

Mild leg exercise is also good. Exercise keeps your calf muscles pumping that blood back to your heart. Walking is good. If you're stuck somewhere, rise and fall on the balls of your feet a half dozen times to tense the calf muscles and get them pumping that blood up. Avoid prolonged periods of sitting or standing still.

Finally, elevating your legs will help defeat gravity by draining the veins of pooled blood and relieving venous pressure. Several times a day, for at least an hour in the morning and an hour in the late afternoon, elevate both legs above your heart.

Pregnant women with vulval varicosities should also follow the three Es of elastic, exercise and elevation. Special elastic crotch supports that compress the labia are available. They help by compressing the veins and preventing a pooling of blood in the varicosities.

Surgery for varicose veins is not considered accepted or routine for pregnant women as it is for others. There are two reasons: one, it could have a deleterious impact on the fetus, and two, it often is not successful because the basic problems—elevated hormone levels and interference with venous blood flow—remain throughout the pregnancy.

I also do not recommend sclerotherapy for pregnant women, primarily because medical researchers have no conclusive evidence about what impact, if any, the chemicals used in the injections have on the fetus.

I do urge pregnant women to take special care with foot hygiene. They should not only wash their feet daily, but make sure to dry between their toes and avoid any infection around the toenails. These damp, dark areas can serve as a point of entry for harmful bacteria. Phlebitis often starts from an insignificant break in the skin in these areas.

After the baby is born, women should wait at least two months before considering surgery or sclerotherapy to see if the symptoms subside.

Menopause

Traditionally, menopause is defined as the time when a woman's reproductive system slows and eventually shuts down. Based on two Greek words meaning "month" and "cease," menopause, or meno-cease, is literally an end to monthly menstrual cycles. It is a gradual, normal process that takes an average of five years to complete, as the ovaries stop releasing eggs and menstrual cycles become irregular and stop. It usually starts for women in their mid-40s and is over by the time they are in their mid-50s.

Over the last 30 years, a more updated definition of menopause has been a "hormonal deficiency disease" that can and should be treated. Not surprisingly, this is a definition promoted by pharmaceutical companies that have just the cure: Hormone Replacement Therapy. This therapy basically consists of taking small doses of estrogen and progestogen, doses even smaller than those contained in most birth control pills. The hormones are prescribed to deal with the discomforts that come with menopause for some, not all, women. These discomforts include hot flashes, vaginal dryness and headaches, and are due to the sharp decline in estrogen that comes with middle age.

There is a growing debate about the wisdom of, and need for, taking these hormones. Proponents of hormone replacement therapy (HRT) argue that treatment relieves a lot of discomforts (which can be fairly severe in some women) and helps women fend off osteoporosis and heart attacks.

Osteoporosis is a loss of bone density that results in brittle bones that break easily, particularly in the hip and spine. The post-menopausal women seem to be at particularly high risk because their estrogen levels drop off then and estrogen is needed to help the bones absorb calcium. The reduction in estrogen also is believed to be why women in their mid-50s become more vulnerable to heart attacks. Estrogen helps keep the arteries of younger women clear by increasing the levels of HDLs—high density lipoproteins—and reducing LDLs—low density lipoproteins. (These are fat carrying proteins which affect the level of cholesterol in our blood.) Opponents of HRT contend that the discomforts of menopause are often exaggerated, and medical intervention is unnecessary. They also insist that the increased risk of endometrial cancer which comes from taking estrogen supplements is far greater than the chance of women having a heart attack or breaking bones because of osteoporosis.

My main concern is the impact that this hormone replacement therapy has on veins, a subject that is not yet getting much media attention. These hormones are being given to women at a time when they seem most susceptible to getting varicose veins. According to a comprehensive study in Switzerland, 48.5% of women who are 45, and 64% of those 55 and older have varicose veins. The mean age for getting varicose veins is 55, just as most women are finished with menopause, their estrogen levels are at their lowest, their lives get more sedentary, their metabolism changes and allows fat deposits to build up in the arteries and their veins are getting old. For more than half a century, their veins have been carrying 4,000 gallons of blood a day. They're a bit tired, deservedly.

When the veins are getting a bit tired, does it make sense to expose them to a burst of estrogen? The question is particularly pertinent now that there is ample research showing that pregnant women experience varicose veins because their bodies have elevated levels of estrogen and progesterone. I'm particularly troubled to see estrogen promoted as a cure for aging as well as the "symptoms" of "hormonal deficiency disease." Women are told that estrogen can help them stay good looking longer by keeping their skin soft and moist and their hair shiny. Apparently they are buying this line: In 1976, according to the Food and Drug Administration, only 1.5 million American women were going through menopause per year, yet 5 million were on estrogen replacement therapy.

There are no comparable figures for 1995. However, there are some recent studies that suggest that younger women are not as quick to take hormone supplements just to, for example, look younger, feel better, and prevent the onset of hot flashes. Further, the Congressional Office of Technology Assessment reported in 1992 that the number of noncontraceptive estrogen prescriptions dropped in the late 1970s as word spread that hormone replacement could lead to endometrial cancer. Also, the Journal of Obstetrics and Gynecology reported in 1995 that the proportion of younger women (those 20–39 years old and not yet near menopause) taking the leading hormone drug, Premarin, dropped from 14% to 8% between 1984 and 1992.

That's the good news. The disturbing news is that the number of prescriptions being issued is growing again as the population ages and women are on hormone replacements for longer and longer periods of time. According to congressional researchers, as of 1990, American doctors wrote more than 30 million prescriptions for noncontraceptive estrogens, surpassing the previous peak achieved in 1975. In 1995, the *Journal of Obstetrics and Gynecology* estimated that as many as one quarter of 36 million menopausal women were currently using some sort of hormonal replacement therapy.

However, congressional researchers report that serious gaps exist in how much doctors know about the effects of taking hormones for long periods of time. Doctors are divided on whether adverse side effects might outweigh good effects, such as protecting women from heart attacks. There is intense pressure for answers from a bipartisan group of women in Congress who have urged that more federal dollars be spent on research in this area.

Meanwhile, some of my colleagues, like Mitchel Goldman, a prominent West Coast specialist in sclerotherapy, believe that estrogen replacement therapy is a principal reason for increased development of varicose veins in midlife.

However, I am also impressed by the research and views of another colleague, Lila Nachtigall, a distinguished endocrinologist at the NYU Medical Center in New York. She sees 20 menopausal women a day and fewer than one per month reports an increase in varicosities as a result of being on hormone replacement therapy.

Nachtigall suggests several reasons:

1. The dose of estrogen is much lower for HRT than that found in oral contraceptives, .0625 mg or less per day vs. 2.5 mg. The lower dose has resulted in HRT's having no adverse effect on the anticlotting factors found in the bloodstream. In her view, HRT estrogen is "quite safe to take even if you have varicose veins," because it will not increase the chance of a clot's forming in the leg.
2. The progesterone used in HRT is different from the one found in oral contraceptives, and the HRT progestogen does not lower HDLs the way the progesterone used in the pill does. (Remember: For a healthy heart, you want your HDLs high and your LDLs low.)
3. Comparatively new transdermal patches that are prescribed in lieu of pills lessen the chance of getting a dangerous leg clot because they bypass the liver, putting hormones directly into the bloodstream. When estrogen is taken orally, the liver releases enzymes that appear to increase the possibility of clots forming. Nachtigall says estrogen supplements "may not be advisable" for women who have a history of thromboemboli or thrombophlebitis because these women are "especially susceptible to clotting" and should not risk "even the most minute effect."

A lot more research needs to be done on this issue, and I'm sure the pressure will increase for answers. At the end of this decade, 21 million American women, the baby boomers, will start turning 50. In no time, we'll have double, then triple, then quadruple the number of women undergoing menopause compared to the 1.5 million experiencing it in 1976. They, along with all women, deserve to know the risks as well as the benefits involved in taking hormone supplements.

Meanwhile, menopausal women who have varicose veins or a family history of varicose veins should discuss the issue with their doctors before starting hormone replacement therapy. If they decide to try it, they should be alert to the symptoms of varicose veins.

Notes

For the discussion on how oral contraceptives work, it's worth taking a moment to read a little refresher course on basic biology: A newborn human female has about 430,000 follicles in her ovaries, each containing the ability to produce an egg. During her reproductive lifetime, only about 400 of these follicles actually release any eggs.

Ovulation, the release of an egg, starts when a follicle ruptures, sending the egg on its way to meet a sperm cell and start a baby. After the egg is released, the follicle collapses. It and the tissue around it develop a yellow pigmentation. This becomes the corpus luteum and this new mass of cells releases the hormone progesterone.

Progesterone tells the pituitary gland to stop releasing hormones that will trigger the release of more eggs. It effectively tells the pituitary: "Stop! One egg is in play. Don't send more until we know if we've got a baby." If the egg is not fertilized in about 14 days, the corpus luteum stops enlarging and disintegrates. If the egg *is* fertilized, the corpus luteum grows for 12 weeks.

Even though the risk of serious side effects has been greater for those who take oral contraceptives, the risk has still been comparatively small. (For example, another English study in 1968 found that deaths from thromboembolic diseases among pill users was 12.1 per 1 million compared to 8.4 for the general population. For more specific studies on the risks involved with oral contraceptives, see the bibliography at the end of this book.)

Getting a clot after surgery does seem more likely for pill users, but taking the pill does not necessarily increase a woman's chance of dying from such a clot.

A 1992 report in the *International Journal of Epidemiology* looks at 60 English and Welsh women under 40 who died from venous thromboembolism in the late 1980s. It found that many had a recent operation or accident that immobilized them, but there was virtually no difference in the percentage of fatalities between those who were taking the pill and those who were not.

The authors suggest that women on the pill could be less vulnerable because oral contraceptives now have lower doses of estrogen and progesterone. However, they also acknowledge that their sample was skewed because it included only young women and only those who died from a thromboembolism, which is not usually fatal among younger women.

Sandra Coney, in a provocative book, *The Menopause Industry*, argues that only 20% of post-menopausal women have a high risk of developing osteoporosis and these women account for only 40% of all fractures. She contends that drug companies interested in promoting HRT have exaggerated osteoporosis as a problem because the hormone supplements help slow the loss of bone density. However, she also reports, the National Osteoporosis Foundation says that if all 50-year-old women with low bone density went on HRT, the lifetime risk of hip fractures for all women would drop only 2% (from 10% to 8%) and spinal fractures 3% (from 25% to 22%).

One 1975 study published in the *New England Journal of Medicine* reported that women using estrogen had a 7.6 times greater risk of endometrial cancer and those at greatest risk used conjugated estrogens for seven years or longer. (Conjugated estrogens are hormones that are synthetically altered to enhance their potency.) A second study at the University of Washington found a 4.5 times greater risk of cancer for women taking estrogen.

However, in the two decades since these studies were done, women on HRT have been taking less estrogen and they are taking it in combination with progestogen. The combination helps lower the risk of endometrial cancer by forcing the uterus to shed its estrogen-fed lining on a monthly basis. Many doctors now feel HRT is safe for most women; however, it does seem that more studies are needed so women and their doctors can weigh the relative risks and benefits of HRT. The need is particularly strong now that (as Coney points out) HRT is no longer being marketed as a short term fix for a short term problem (hot flashes); now it's billed as a multi-year fix for a lot of problems (heart conditions, osteoporosis and the general problems of aging).

Sales dropped off in the late 1970s after doctors reported higher instances of endometrial and breast cancer for those taking estrogen, but they climbed back up again as drug companies refocused the debate on how HRT can prevent osteoporosis and heart attacks. It's estimated that 30% of the post menopausal women in America now use HRT.

Among the many studies cited in this chapter are two worth mentioning here. One was published in the July 1963 *American Journal of Obstetrics and Gynecology* entitled "Venous distensibility during the menstrual cycle" by A.M. McCausland, Frances Holmes and Alfred D. Trotter, Jr. The second, entitled "Oral Contraception: Past, Present and Future Perspectives," was written by Daniel R. Mishell in the March 1992 edition of the *International Journal of Fertility*. Also, the definitive study showing how women get varicose veins far more frequently than men was the *Basle Study III* cited at the end of Chapter 3.

Two books mentioned in this chapter are John Camp's *Magic, Myth and Medicine* (Taplinger Publishing, 1974) and *Estrogen: The Facts Can Change Your Life* by Lila Nachtigall and Joan Rattner Heilman (The Body Press, 1986).

CHAPTER 8

■■■■■■■■■■■■■■■■■■■■■■■■■■■■■■■■

VITAMINS

Earlier in this book, a high-fiber diet was mentioned as one possible way of avoiding, or delaying the onset of, varicose veins. I want to expand a bit now on the issues of nutrition and vitamins and how they might have an impact on veins. Patients frequently ask me: Can vitamins help me avoid or cure varicose veins?

First, allow me to answer that basic question with one big shrug. Doctors don't know for sure how effective vitamin supplements are for such health problems as varicose veins, breast cancer or arteriosclerosis. Scientists don't even agree on the minimum amount of each vitamin we need each day to stay healthy.

As of this writing, the U.S. Food and Drug Administration has decreed that only two dietary supplements—calcium and folic acid—can make curative claims. These are the only two supplements that have met the stiff standard of having "significant scientific agreement" among qualified experts on their claims to help avoid osteoporosis and the risk of neural tube birth defects, respectively. Serious research on the question of how dietary supplements work has only recently been undertaken and it will be years before there are any definitive answers.

To understand the vitamin controversy and evaluate its importance to you as a consumer, you must know some facts about vitamins and how they generally interact with your body. Vitamins are organic compounds composed of carbon, hydrogen, oxygen and sometimes nitrogen. The difference between one vitamin and another is the way these compounds are arranged. We all need vitamins in small amounts for normal growth and good health. By working in conjuction with fats, carbohydrates and proteins in the blood, they transform foods into energy, but they do not by themselves provide energy. If you are dieting and think vitamins will restore your energy levels, think again. Vitamins need some food to work properly.

Some vitamins are more helpful to some body parts than others because tissues and organs differ in composition and thus in nutritional requirements. The absence of one particular vitamin is like absenteeism in a factory: Sometimes a job simply does not get done, other times the end product is defective. Diseases form when cells are inadequately nourished and the food we ingest is not properly utilized.

Vitamin deficiencies are found in all generations—the newborn and very young, adolescents, pregnant women, the elderly. Supplements are now routine for many of us. This is because gradually, over the last 400 years, scientists have slowly figured out that vitamin deficiencies cause specific diseases and they contend that supplements can cure or prevent the onset of these diseases.

The earliest hint that a vitamin deficiency could cause a disease comes from accounts of how an Elizabethan seaman, Sir James Lancaster, fought scurvy (bleeding gums) in 1601 by introducing fruit juices into his ship's diet. Lancaster's theory was revived by James Lind in 1757 and Captain Cook in 1772. A Japanese admiral, K. Takaki, in 1881, wiped out beriberi (another vitamin deficiency disease which damages the nerves and produces numbness in the hands and feet) by improving the crew's diet. The notion that there were certain "accessory substances or accessory food factors" (later called vitamins) that are essential for our body to get adequate nutrition was suggested by Sir Frederick Hopkins in 1906.

The original form of the word vitamin took shape in 1912 when a Polish biochemist, Casimir Funk, contended that there were four "vitamines" needed to fight scurvy, rickets (bowed legs), beriberi and pellagra (a combination of skin, gastrointestinal and nerve disorders). His word "vitamine" came from the Latin "vita" (life) and "amine" which are chemical components or building blocks derived from proteins that cannot be manufactured by the body and are essential for life. By 1920, scientists had discovered some vitamins that were not truly "vital amines" and coined a term for the entire group of "accessory substances" by combining the words and calling them "vitamins."

There are 13 vitamins, each having a letter identification because that's the way scientists in the first half of this century chose to distinguish them. Later, when one vitamin was found to be many different substances, numbers were added. Then, some numbers were dropped when those vitamins were found to be unnecessary for humans.

Some vitamins, like A, D, E and K, are oil, or fat, soluble; that is, they get stored in the body for long periods of time, even indefinitely. When you take more of these vitamins than the recommended daily allotment, you can in effect poison yourself. Other vitamins, like B and C, are water soluble, which means excess amounts are washed out of the body through the kidneys or intestines.

Vitamins perform a variety of tasks. Vitamin A is needed for new cell growth and healthy tissue. Folic acid, a form of vitamin B, helps the body manufacture red blood cells. Vitamin C promotes growth and tissue repair. Vitamin D helps the body absorb calcium and phosphorus in bone formation. Vitamin K is essential in getting blood to clot. Vitamin E is a preservative and anti-oxidant that helps other compounds, like vitamin A, do their job by preventing oxygen from destroying them.

Scientists know these basic facts about vitamins and yet they don't know, for example, how vitamins interact with one another, or how much of any particular vitamin the human body actually needs.

The League of Nations (predecessor to the United Nations) took a big step in trying to answer these questions in 1936 when it set a minimum standard for the entire world by publishing internationally agreed upon standards for daily vitamin requirements. The League said then, for example, that an adult needs 3,000 international units (a standard of measurement) of vitamin A per day, 300 IUs of vitamin B1, 30 milligrams of vitamin C and 500 IUs of vitamin D. Many countries still stick to those standards. In the United States, those figures are considered a bit low in some categories. For example, the FDA's standards for vitamin A and C consumption are 5,000 IUs and 60 mg per day, respectively. The current U.S. standards grew out of a 1969 White House Conference on Food, Nutrition and Health which tried to address deficiencies in the American diet by proposing that the federal government develop a system for identifying the nutritional qualities of food.

The U.S. Food and Drug Administration has been trying to perform that task ever since in a way that satisfies both experts in nutrition and big business interests who would like to be able to call everything "lite," "high fiber," "fat free," and "nutritious" without necessarily having to prove it. For 20 years, the FDA promoted something called the U.S. RDAs (Recommended Daily Allowances), which were the approximate amounts of vitamins, minerals and protein that it thought people need to stay healthy. (The U.S. RDAs were based on other RDAs—which stood for Recommended Dietary Allowances—suggested in 1968 by the National Academy of Sciences' Food and Nutrition Board.)

By the summer of 1994, a whole new set of FDA regulations took effect. Gone are the U.S. RDAs. Now we have DVs, DRVs and RDIs.

DVs are Daily Values. These values refer to the nutritional value of food and are roughly the amounts that the FDA thinks anyone over the age of four needs to stay healthy. You won't necessarily die faster or catch beriberi if you don't get all these DVs in your diet; they serve as a guide, a rule of thumb based on a 2,000-calorie daily diet (which is too much for some people and too little for others).

DVs are also supposed to guide food producers to help them be more truthful when they advertise and label their products. They can't call something "high fiber," for example, unless the product provides at least 20% of someone's daily fiber requirement. Take a look at that box of cereal in your kitchen. Today the label probably says "rich in fiber" (vs. "high fiber") because it provides only 18% of the daily requirement and that's the most the manufacturer can claim.

DVs are like an umbrella over two other terms that the FDA put into orbit as a result of 1990 legislation: DRVs and RDIs. DRVs are Daily Reference Values, which set recommended limits on potentially harmful foodstuffs that never had standards before, like fat, cholesterol, potassium and sodium.

RDIs are Reference Daily Intakes. They replace U.S. RDAs. They give consumers a rough idea of how much of the various vitamins and minerals they might want to consume daily to stay healthy. These suggested limits are based on a 1968 study by the National Academy of Sciences. In 1994, however, the FDA stated that these limits may be revised to account for new research that suggests that some of the vitamin supplement doses recommended then are too high or too low.

The charts at the end of this chapter give you the DRVs and RDIs. As you study them, remember that they are based on a 2,000-calorie-a-day diet. The very young (ages four to six) and those over 51 need a bit less; male contruction workers between the ages of 25 and

50 might need as many as 4,000 calories a day (depending on whether they're doing the heavy lifting or directing traffic at the construction site). Thus, we're providing a third chart, also from the FDA, which provides the recommended caloric intake based on your age, sex and activity level.

Now that you know a little something about the recommended daily intake of vitamins and minerals and a tiny bit about how they work, you might wonder what happens to your arteries and veins if you add a few here and there to your diet.

First, a warning. Don't get carried away with the pages you are about to read. This is one field where a little common sense goes a long way—physically and emotionally. For good physical health, your body needs only tiny amounts of vitamins. One ounce of vitamin B12 can supply the daily requirements for more than four million people. Too much of a good thing can and will hurt you. It's estimated that 2,000 children a year in the U.S. are poisoned by taking their mothers' prenatal iron supplements. Other people, grownups, overdose on vitamins all the time and often they don't realize it because they take *more* vitamin and mineral supplements to deal with the problems created by the first overdose.

Emotionally, you can overdose on vitamins by believing all the claims that the manufacturers, and some scientists, make about their curative and preventive properties. Just remember, however, that so far, the FDA is only allowing these claims for calcium and folic acid. The claims cited below need further proof before they are widely accepted.

It now appears that some vitamins—notably B6, A and C—are particularly important for healthy arteries and veins. I'm not suggesting you take supplements, but rather noting that there is some interesting research worth knowing if you have varicose veins, phlebitis or any cardiovascular disease.

Vitamin B6, also known as pyridoxine, was first identified in 1934 by Dr. Paul Gyorgy and first manufactured synthetically in 1939. There is now a consensus in the medical community that B6 is needed for amino acids to work effectively in the body. B6 also plays all sorts of roles in how the body metabolizes fats.

In terms of vascular disorders, some research now suggests that B6 might reduce the buildup of homocysteine in the blood. Homocysteine is a chemical that seems to accelerate the formation of arteriosclerotic plaques that clog our arteries. Some years ago, researchers at the University of California School of Medicine in San Francisco noted that monkeys deprived of B6 in their high cholesterol diets developed a typical arteriosclerotic lesion, or clot, in their arteries. The experiments were repeated at other research facilities on dogs and chickens and the results were the same. Then, when these animals were given B6 supplements, along with a high cholesterol diet, no lesions developed. Thus scientists believe that extra B6 in the diet somehow disposes of the surplus cholesterol.

We know that B6 is needed for our bodies to get full use of proteins and carbohydrates. Some recent research suggests that as fat consumption increases in our diets, more B6 is needed. Some researchers consider arteriosclerosis as a modern day deficiency disease due to a shortage of B6 in an otherwise high-fat diet.

The current RDI for vitamin B6 is 2 mg per day, the same as it's been for over 20 years. The amount is more than most people ordinarily consume even though the vitamin is widely available in foods like beef liver, pork products, veal, fresh fish, bananas, cabbage, avocados, peanuts, walnuts, raisins, prunes, cereal grain and grapes. You might wonder how we develop a B6 deficiency when we know the amount we need and the vitamin is available in so many foods. One possible answer is that some people seem to be more dependent on vitamin B6 than others because of the way that their metabolism digests food and translates it into energy. Another is that our diets keep changing. For example, anyone with high cholesterol levels can tell you that beef liver, pork, veal and avocados, all rich in B6, are also high in fat content and they are advised not to eat them. Fresh fish and grapes are expensive and not always available. Bread—without butter—and cereal—with skim milk—are acceptable for someone fighting to trim cholesterol levels, but these foods don't have as much B6 as they used to have because it gets lost when the grains are milled into flour.

The vitamin loss caused by the milling process is well known. That's why we have so much "vitamin enriched" flour and bread on supermarket shelves: Manufacturers have restored thiamine, niacin, riboflavin (all members of the vitamin B water soluble group) to the flour after it was lost in milling. However, vitamin B6, which is expensive, got lost and is not restored by manufacturers. Therefore a typical diet does tend to supply insufficient B6.

Vitamin A was first clearly recognized as a vitamin in 1913 by Professor Paul Karrer, who was awarded the Nobel Prize for his work. A fat soluble vitamin, vitamin A is naturally present in fish and fish liver oils, butter and the liver fat of various animals. Vegetables and fruits contain one class of pigments called carotenoid pigments that are converted to vitamin A in the body. One of these pigments, carotene, is a good source of this vitamin. One major function of vitamin A is to help produce antibodies, white blood cells and the mucus that lines body cavities and helps keep them cleansed and free of bacteria.

Vitamin A also helps to maintain endothelial tissues, the membranes that form the innermost lining of our veins and arteries. The theory is that inadequate "feeding" of these blood vessels, as the result of a vitamin A deficiency for example, causes the vessels to stiffen and harden, creating an ideal platform for the formation of arteriosclerotic plaques, and even blood clots, within the veins.

Vitamin A is clearly one of the most controversial vitamins. Scientists disagree vehemently about its merits and demerits. Just be aware that vitamin A, like vitamin D, can be toxic if you take too much of it. Even though they are sold without a prescription, vitamin A supplements should be taken only under a doctor's direction with a prescribed daily dose.

As a practicing vascular surgeon, I know from clinical experience that vitamin C is essential for the proper healing of injured tissue and necessary for combating infections. Medical research supports these observations as well. Vitamin C does more than prevent scurvy. It also appears now that it helps control cholesterol levels in the bloodstream and helps to heal injured vein and artery walls.

A variety of studies over the past four decades show that those who take vitamin C supplements of one-half to one full gram per day can cut cholesterol levels by as much as 30%. Some studies focused on smokers have suggested that they might be more prone to cardiovascular diseases because their vitamin C levels are lower than non-smokers'.

Vitamin C also seems to keep the interior walls of veins and arteries healthy by helping them heal when they are injured or their shape is altered (for example, when they are expanded during pregnancy).

Vitamin E is by far one of the most controversial of the 13 vitamins. Much has been written about the theoretical benefit it has on circulatory diseases, particularly intermittent claudication, a term used when someone consistently gets leg pains after repeatedly walking the same distance. As recently as 1993, two studies in Boston suggested that vitamin E's antioxidant properties prevent the oxidation of fatty acids in cell membranes and in the low-density lipoprotein (LDLs), the main carrier of cholesterol in the blood. One hundred twenty thousand men and women were followed in these studies. Those who took 100 IUs of vitamin E a day for at least two years were 40% less likely to develop heart disease.

While the most recent studies are interesting (and on a scale that is large enough to be significant), I don't think there is any convincing evidence at present that vitamin E can prevent or cure varicose veins or their complications.

After all, there are also studies which show that garlic extracts seem to cut blood cholesterol levels by lowering LDLs and raising HDLs (high-density lipoproteins). This means garlic supplements, like vitamin E, could help reduce the risk of heart attacks. Other studies suggest garlic can help prevent stomach and other forms of cancer.

Extracts of garlic and onions also have antibacterial and antifungal properties which can inhibit blood platelets from coming together to form a clot. This means that extracts of garlic and onion might prevent blood clots and help those with varicose veins avoid the serious problems of thrombophlebitis.

As noted above, doctors' suspicions are not facts. However, I also realize that millions of Americans are not waiting for the FDA or scientists to come up with facts. They are taking vitamins on faith.

A 1993 *Newsweek* poll showed that 70% of all Americans have used some vitamin supplements at least occasionally and 15% of the daily users started within the last year. Those statistics undoubtedly brought smiles to the faces of executives in an industry that has annual gross sales of an estimated $3.3 billion. So, when patients ask me if vitamins could help, I try to give them some of the background above and caution them not to expect miracles. I also tell them that I find some of the research on vitamin C to be particularly compelling and so I generally prescribe vitamin C supplements for patients after surgery. I believe it helps them heal faster. Like chicken soup, a little vitamin C can't hurt. However, we are a long way from the time when a vitamin pill a day will keep the doctor away.

DAILY REFERENCE VALUES (DRVS)*

Food Component	DRV
fat	65 grams (g)
saturated fatty acids	20 g
cholesterol	300 milligrams (mg)
total carbohydrate	300 g
fiber	25 g
sodium	2,400 mg
potassium	3,500 mg
protein**	50 g

* Based on 2,000 calories a day for adults and children over 4 only
** DRV for protein does not apply to certain populations. Reference Daily Intake (RDI) for protein has been established for these groups: children 1 to 4 years: 16 g; infants under 1 year: 14 g; pregnant women: 60 g; nursing mothers: 65 g.

REFERENCE DAILY INTAKES (RDIS)*

Nurtrient	Amount
Vitamin A	5,000 International Units (IU)
Vitamin C	60 milligrams (mg)
Thiamin	1.5 mg
Riboflavin	1.7 mg
Niacin	20 mg
Calcium	1.0 grams (g)
Iron	18 mg
Vitamin D	400 IU
Vitamin E	30 IU
Vitamin B6	2.0 mg
Folic acid	0.4 mg
Vitamin B12	6 micrograms (mcg)
Phosphorus	1.0 g
Iodine	150 mcg
Magnesium	400 mg
Zinc	15 mg
Copper	2 mg
Biotin	0.3 mg
Pantothenic acid	10 mg

*Based on National Academy of Science's 1968 Recommended Dietary Allowances

| RECOMMENDED ENERGY INTAKE* | | |
| Calories Per Day | | |
Light Activity	Moderate Activity	Heavy Activity
Children		
4–6	1,800	
7–10	2,000	
Men		
11–14	2,500	
15–18	3,000	
19–24	2,700	3,000	3,600
25–50	3,000	3,200	4,000
51+		2,300*	
Women		
11–18	2,200	
19–24	2,000	2,100	2,600
25–50	2,200	2,300	2,800
51+		1,900*	

*Based on light to moderate activity. Pregnant women in their second and third trimesters should add 300 calories to the figures the table indicates for their age. Nursing mothers should add 500.

Notes

Some of the research that suggests B6 helps to fight clots was done by Doctors Edward Gruberg and Stephen Raymond. In their 1981 book, *Vitamin B6, Arteriosclerosis And Your Heart,* they said B6 helps prevent hardening of the arteries by cleansing homocysteine from your body.

Two significant studies at the Harvard School of Public Health and Brigham and Women's Hospital in Boston concluded in 1992 that vitamin E could help prevent heart attacks. Dr. Meir Stampfer reported at the American Heart Association's annual meeting in November of that year that of 87,245 nurses studied across the U.S., 17% took vitamin E and those taking E supplements for more than two years had a 46% lower risk of getting a heart attack. In a companion study of 51,529 male health professionals, Dr. Eric Rimm said that men who took vitamin E had a 37% lower risk of heart disease. The minimum dose used was 100 international units per day.

As appealing as this news is to those who fear a heart attack, those who are taking an anticoagulant for thrombophlebitis or other reasons should be wary of vitamin E because it can interfere with blood clotting in people with certain medical problems and thus increase the risk of hemorrhagic stroke.

Dr. Alton Ochsner, formerly professor and chairman of the department of surgery at Tulane Medical School, was one of the first to point out the importance of vitamin C in the diet as a healing agent. Many recent studies have debated the issue of whether vitamin C also helps to fight cancer, but in my practice, I see more of its healing properties.

CHAPTER 9

∎∎∎∎∎∎∎∎∎∎∎∎∎∎∎∎∎∎∎∎∎∎∎∎∎∎∎∎∎∎∎

LOOKING AHEAD

Our closing chapter refers to the advice we have given in this book about things you can do to control your own future and avoid varicose veins and their dangerous complications. We also wish to speculate a bit on what advances medicine might (or should) make by the millennium in terms of treating, finding a definitive cause for and preventing varicose veins.

It sounds simple, but our basic advice for preventing varicose veins has been:

(1) Exercise;
(2) Eat right (meaning a high fiber diet and not too much food in general);
(3) Avoid prolonged periods of standing and sitting (or if you can't avoid them, exercise your legs frequently during these periods);
(4) Keep your clothing loose (especially in the thigh and groin area); and,
(5) Take good care of your feet, making sure that they're free of infections and ingrown nails.

There is no guarantee that these prophylactic measures will stop varicose veins from appearing if you have a tendency toward them. As we pointed out earlier, your genetic makeup has a lot to do with whether or not you will get them.

According to a 1994 study in France of men and women in their 30s: "The risk of developing varicose veins was 90% when both parents suffered from the disease, 25% in males and 62% in females when one parent was affected and 20% when neither parent was affected."

Heredity is not the entire story. Since environmental factors can be controlled to a certain extent, it is possible for you to forestall the appearance of these blue snakes, or at least minimize or avoid the complications that so often come with them.

In the next 10 years, expect to see vascular surgeons finding new ways to preserve the saphenous vein for other purposes like bypass surgery.

One promising technique pioneered by this author involves putting a plastic band around the exterior of the saphenous vein at the point where a valve inside is not working properly. This band forces the valve doors to close as they are designed to do, preventing the damaging backflow that causes the vein below to bulge out in varicosities. The surgeon then makes tiny incisions over the varicosities to remove the unsightly sections of the vein.

This banding technique is not good for everyone. For example, if the cusps or doors on your valve are destroyed or missing, banding won't work and your surgeon will have to remove a larger portion of the saphenous vein. (Don't worry if the entire vein has to be removed and you might need bypass surgery down the road. There are 24 other suitable conduits in your body for bypass surgery.)

Another technique pioneered by Donald Kistner, a vascular surgeon in Hawaii, involves opening the saphenous vein surgically and exposing the valve cusp so that it can be repaired.

These procedures are effective when your vein valves are malfunctioning. However, if there are other causes, such as weak vein walls, then these measures won't work. When the vein valves are beyond repair, surgeons are starting to harvest vein valves from the arm to put them in the saphenous or deep veins in the leg. This technique has proved to be especially useful for those patients who have special problems like venous ulcers and venous hypertension in the leg veins.

It might take longer for these surgical advances and others to become widely used because insurance companies increasingly do not want to pay for the extensive diagnostic tests needed to identify problems such as a malfunctioning vein valve. They also don't want to pay for the slightly longer hospital confinements that are associated with them. These limitations are a problem particularly for my patients who are enrolled in a health maintenance group.

Patients who have had a pulmonary embolus, or who are at risk of having one, can expect to see new devices or refinement of existing ones that block the passage of blood clots through the vena cava. The most widely used device is still the Greenfield caval filter but even that one has been refined several times in the last decade. Undoubtedly, we will see even more improvements in this filter technology.

You also might see more and more people having these filters inserted, particularly the elderly, since many of them require a blood thinning drug to avoid the formation of clots in the leg veins and its most serious complication, a pulmonary embolus. Doctors are now finding that many of these patients (according to one study, 38% of those on a therapeutic dose of Coumarin) have experienced a minor or major hemorrhage because of the drug. The filters are more expensive than drug therapy to install initially, but they save money in the long run because they avoid costly, prolonged hospitalization for treatment of hemorrhages.

Although the medical community understands that early surgical treatment of varicosities prevents nasty complications that ultimately develop if varicose veins are ignored, insurance companies still resist paying for the surgery and thus we have one million Americans today who are suffering with varicose ulcers.

One of the more unpleasant complications that come with venous insufficiency are severely swollen legs. Some doctors are experimenting with drugs that seem to give some relief, but the results are far from conclusive and the side effects are unclear.

As we look forward to the turn of the century and understand that controlling the growth of medical expenses is a national priority, you can expect to see a fight shaping up over spider veins. Already, a growing number of insurance companies resist paying for treatment, arguing that it is being done purely for cosmetic purposes. In some cases that's true, but spider veins are often quite painful and can signal the existence of otherwise invisible, but potentially serious, varicose veins. Removing them with sclerotherapy makes the patient feel better in the short run, and it also removes the site for a potential complication later on, like the development of an ulcer or a blood clot.

The insurance companies aside, doctors are now testing a new generation of sclerosing solutions that when injected under the skin cause less pain and are less prone to leave a disfiguring pigment stain. Expect to see some of these come into mainstream use before the decade is over.

In terms of finding the ultimate causes for varicose veins, you can expect to see more research into the role of genetics. This research could result in a new kind of treatment for varicose veins: gene therapy. However, that's probably more than a decade away.

You also will probably hear about more research into the impact that our sex hormones have on the cardiovascular system. We are just now beginning to appreciate the impact that they have on the vascular system. As this research develops, we might find that some people should not be on a hormone replacement therapy because it triggers problems in otherwise quiescent varicose veins. Others might have no problems taking hormone supplements. In fact, hormone supplements might help some people by keeping the inner lining of the veins healthy. The picture, as of this writing, is unclear.

You can also expect to see more research on the impact that vitamin and other dietary supplements have on our circulatory system. Are varicose veins caused by some vitamin deficiencies? Is diet a factor that makes varicose veins more common in some cultures than others?

Obviously, you cannot and should not wait for answers to these and other questions. As we mentioned above, there are some rules to follow if you want to delay the onset of varicose veins or alleviate the symptoms.

Avoid, whenever possible, long periods of standing or sitting. If you must stand on a line or sit for a long period of time, make a conscious effort to flex the muscles of your leg. Wiggle your toes frequently. Slowly raise and lower yourself on the balls of your feet.

It is also a good idea to break up the inactivity (and monotony) of a long trip by walking for several minutes every hour or two. If you are on an airplane or train ride that stretches beyond several hours, walk up and down the aisle at least once an hour.

The chair, one of our most common conveniences, is a terrible invention of civilization—at least as far as our veins are concerned. It started with the ancient Egyptians and they too had varicose veins. While it makes sitting comfortable, it increases the pressure on the leg veins and leads to a damaging habit: crossing your legs.

If your legs are crossed right now, uncross them and try to break the habit. Crossed legs increase the pressure within the leg veins. While we do not know if sitting or crossing our legs actually causes varicose veins, we do know that prolonged sitting will aggravate an existing tendency toward varicose veins.

Eat properly. Doctors will tell you that they see very fat patients, and they see very old patients, but rarely do they see very old fat patients. Obesity and long life are not compatible. A proper diet not only reduces pressure in your leg veins; it also could prolong your life. Your diet must include lots of fiber, fresh fruits and vegetables, water and protein. All of these substances help keep your bowels moving with regularity. The correlation between constipation and varicose veins is twofold: One, a full colon puts pressure on the veins that run along the back of the abdominal cavity, slowing the return flow of blood from veins in the leg. This increased pressure is passed along to the leg veins. A high fiber diet will keep the colon empty and the extra pressure off the legs. Two, sitting too long on a toilet seat puts undue pressure on the thigh veins and is worse than sitting on a chair. The only thing that's worse, perhaps, is straining during defecation. This feature of constipation puts pressure on the abdominal veins, which in turn puts pressure on the leg veins.

Wear loose clothing. Although we insist on looking good, no matter how uncomfortable it makes us feel, clothing that is too tight contricts the flow of blood in the veins just beneath the skin. Such items as calf-length boots (no longer in vogue but always threatening to reappear), pantyhose that are overly tight at the groin and stuffed-sausage girdles or corsets that strangle the upper thighs are a case in point. I truly wonder sometimes if we would have a lower incidence of varicose veins if we adopted the loose fitting garments of the Third World where varicose veins are relatively rare. I refer, of course, to the sari of India, the kenhga of East Africa and even the stola of ancient Rome.

Keep your feet in good shape. Americans think feet are funny; they don't take them seriously at all. However, foot problems are not only uncomfortable, they also can be dangerous. First, keep them clean. Advertisements promote clean faces, clean necks, clean fingernails, clean teeth and (the all time biggie) clean armpits. But did you ever see a television commercial hawking clean feet? However offensive, no one ever died from an underarm odor, but the consequences of dirty feet can be fatal. Dirty feet can lead to phlebitis or blood clots in the leg veins. A fatal pulmonary embolus can start from a neglected skin erosion in the foot that is attached to a leg with varicose veins.

Even athlete's foot, a fungus infection, can lead to an inflammation of a leg vein and other problems. An ingrown toenail also can cause a serious infection that can lead to gangrene of the foot and its amputation. Therefore, clip toenails at least twice a month. Do it in good light, cutting straight across, even with the tip of the toe. File any sharp edges with an emery board. Better yet, let your podiatrist do it if you have difficulty reaching your feet.

Never consider a foot or leg injury minor. Do not ignore or neglect it. An open wound in the leg or foot should be treated promptly. Remember that your feet are encased in a dark, moist atmosphere most of the day, the perfect environment for bacteria to grow. So keep your feet not only clean, but dry and supple. Creams and powders are useful. Dry, scaly feet should be moistened with pure lanolin preparations applied smoothly and evenly. Sweaty feet promote fungal infections. An antifungal agent massaged on the foot or sprinkled in shoes can help fight fungus.

One last bit of advice to young women who do not have varicose veins but who fear them because of a family history. Don't let your fears immobilize you. Remember that varicose veins sometimes skip generations. Also, there are many women without varicose veins who have borne many children and there are women who have never been pregnant and yet they suffer with varicose veins.

If you have a family history of varicose veins and get them during pregnancy, treat yourself well. Exercise. Elevate your legs daily. Don't gain too much weight. And remember that they will largely disappear after you give birth.

Notes

The 1994 French study cited here appeared in the *Journal of Dermatology, Surgery and Oncology*. Entitled "Importance of the Familial Factor in Varicose Disease," it was written by Andre Cornu-Thenard, Pierre Boivin, Jean-Michel Baud, Isabelle De Vincenzi and Patrick Carpentier.

CHAPTER 10

∎∎∎∎∎∎∎∎∎∎∎∎∎∎∎∎∎∎∎∎∎∎∎∎∎∎∎∎∎∎∎

MOST COMMON
QUESTIONS

What are varicose veins?
Varicose veins are malformed, defective blood vessels that have lost their elasticity. They have become stretched out of shape beyond normal length and width, and they appear enlarged, tortuous and discolored. They get this way when vein valves in the legs are missing or malfunction for some reason. When the valves don't work properly, blood in the veins backs up, pools and presses against vein walls. As a result, veins lose their shape, and serious complications can ensue.

What do varicose veins look like?
Varicose veins vary greatly from individual to individual and from leg to leg in terms of their severity and appearance. Some are invisible to the eye. Others are bulging knotted blue cords on the legs. There is often little correlation between the severity of the symptoms and the extent of the varicosities.

How common are varicose veins?
Varicose veins are one of the most common vascular diseases in Western cultures. By some estimates, one-third of the population is affected. The number of people with varicose veins increases with age and it affects women more than men. One authoritative study found 8% of women under 25 affected compared with 64% of those 55 and older.

How can I tell if I have varicose veins?
The most common symptoms are a dull aching or tired feeling and a feeling of fullness in the legs when standing or sitting for long periods of time. Often, the symptoms get worse toward the end of the day. Usually, the aching or tiredness in the legs cannot be pinpointed. Generally, if these symptoms go away when you elevate

your legs, varicose veins are the problem—unless proven otherwise. However, be wary of blaming all your symptoms on a few varicosities. There may be other causes.

Are leg cramps that come in the middle of the night another sign?
Varicose veins can cause night cramps, otherwise known as charley horse. They occur most frequently in the calf muscles and can be severe enough to wake you. You will experience them most often after a day of prolonged sitting or standing.

Where do varicose veins commonly occur?
Usually they are found in the superficial veins in your legs, just under your skin. The vein most frequently affected is the saphenous vein, which runs along the inside of your leg from the ankle to the groin.

Are they hereditary?
Probably. Doctors who treat varicose veins have noticed for years that their patients often have someone in the family—a mother, father, aunt or uncle—with this problem. Now scientists believe they have isolated the gene that causes varicose veins.

It is unclear if the gene causes people to have defective vein valves or vein walls. These theories are explained in detail in Chapter 3. Ultimately, the discovery could lead to gene therapy as one way to treat varicose veins, but it is not an option available to patients today.

Does pregnancy cause varicose veins?
Pregnancy does not cause varicose veins, but it can be a contributing factor by triggering varicosities in someone who is predisposed to getting them (for example, those who were born with defective vein valves). Doctors make this distinction because they know that many pregnant women have no problem with varicose veins. Others don't get varicose veins until their fourth or fifth or tenth child is born. And many get varicose veins during pregnancy, only to see them disappear after they give birth.

Pregnancy is believed to be a contributing factor because it causes a surge in the level of female hormones, estrogen and progesterone, in a woman's body. These hormones in large doses soften the vein wall, making it harder for those vein valves to close tight.

Are there other causes?
I believe there are many cultural factors that contribute to the high incidence of varicose veins in Western societies. For example, we

spend a lot of time sitting in chairs. From grammar school through college, we spend at least 40 hours a week sitting (assuming five hours a day sitting in school, three hours a night for homework and TV, multiplied by five days a week). This schedule goes on for 10 months of the year for 17 years. Then we go to office-based jobs for more sitting. All this sitting puts pressure on the veins in the back of our legs and results in less use of calf muscles that are so important for propelling blood back to the heart.

Another cultural factor is diet. Urbanized Western societies tend to eat low fiber diets. This diet causes hard stools and more frequent constipation. When a person must strain to pass his stool, he puts undue pressure on the abdominal muscles. The pressure is transmitted to the major leg veins, causing them to dilate and make vein valves incompetent.

Why do varicose veins affect older people more, especially women?
The short answer is that their systems have experienced more wear and tear, and sooner or later, something gives. I do believe, however, that there are several other reasons why older women get varicose veins more frequently than younger women and men. For one thing, because women live longer than men, there are more elderly women than elderly men and they have more time for their veins to malfunction.

A second reason: Prior pregnancies, a factor that doesn't affect men. Even if their varicose veins disappeared after giving birth, women who experienced them during pregnancy have had an experience that stretched their veins beyond the norm. As we age, the muscles throughout our body, including muscles in the walls of our veins, lose their elasticity. Veins already stretched once by pregnancy will stretch a bit more when they're older.

A third reason: The increasing popularity over the last 30 years of hormone replacement therapy for women in menopause. There's no doubt that estrogen supplements can help keep women comfortable, prettier and in overall better spirits through their menopausal years. There's also some evidence now that the supplements might help prevent heart attacks and stem bone loss due to osteoporosis. (See Chapter 7.) However, I think they can also soften the vein walls, just as elevated levels of estrogen and progesterone have this effect during pregnancy. This side effect means the vein walls are softened at a time when their elasticity is waning anyway with age. Much more research needs to be done on this subject.

Are there different kinds of varicose veins?
Yes. Varicose veins are divided into two major groups. The most common are primary varicose veins, those inherited from family genes. The second type are acquired varicose veins. These occur after your leg is injured and a vein wall is damaged by the formation of a clot or thrombosis. As the clot moves through the vein, it destroys the vein valves and secondary varicose veins form.

Are spider veins also varicose veins?
Spider veins show up as a collection of tiny red or purple lines around your knees or ankles. (Sometimes they're even found around your nose.) They are not really varicose veins, which by definition are veins that are stretched beyond their normal length and dilated beyond their normal diameter. Spider veins are slightly enlarged venules (those veins which connect capillaries with large veins) and they are located close to skin surface.

Spider veins are thought to be influenced by the female hormones and can appear more prominent on women taking oral contraceptives. They also can be triggered by varicosities that may be invisible. Insurance companies think spider veins are harmless and they are increasingly unwilling to pay for their treatment, arguing that women with spider veins seek treatment for cosmetic reasons. However, women with spider veins often report symptoms that are very much like those for varicose veins.

How do you treat varicose veins?
The treatment depends on the severity of the problem. If the symptoms are not too severe, the first course of action is the Three Es: elastic, exercise and elevation. (See Chapter 5 for a full explanation of all treatment options.) If these actions don't work well enough, diseased veins can be removed surgically. Another, more experimental surgical procedure involves banding, which is wrapping a plastic band around the outside of the diseased vein at a point where the vein valve is not closing properly. Finally, for those seeking to treat spider veins or residual varicose veins, there is sclerotherapy, which involves injecting a chemical into the vein, causing a clot to form and adhere to the vein wall and forcing blood to find another path back to the heart.

What are the risks involved with these treatments?
The main risk involved with the Three Es is that they won't work. As for surgery, the operation for removing part of a diseased vein is now done on an outpatient basis by most vascular surgeons. You're in and out of the hospital in a day, without an overnight stay, and often the surgery is done under local anesthesia. The risks with banding are unclear because the procedure is so new. As for sclerotherapy, the main risk is that the chemical injected could leave a slight stain under the skin that won't disappear for months, if ever.

Can varicose veins recur after surgery?
If your varicose veins have been removed, they cannot recur. However, sometimes varicosities pop up after surgery in a vein not initially affected or in small veins where problems were invisible prior to the operation. Varicosities after surgery develop because your blood has to find alternate paths back to the heart after a vein is removed. The increased volume of blood in these residual veins causes them to dilate, and voilà! a new problem. These new varicosities, however, are usually tiny and can be treated with sclerotherapy in your doctor's office.

What are the possible complications from varicose veins?
The most common complications are phlebitis or thrombophlebitis. Other, more serious complications include leg ulcers, permanently swollen legs and pulmonary emboli or blood clots to the lung. (See Chapter 6 for more details.)

Can varicose veins be prevented?
It is virtually impossible to avoid varicose veins if you have that family gene. However, there are things you can do to delay the onset, soften the impact and generally avoid complications from developing.

Try to avoid prolonged periods of standing or sitting. If you have a choice in jobs between one that has you sitting all day and one that lets you move around a lot, take the latter. If you have to take long train or plane rides, make sure you get up and walk down the aisle every hour or so. On long car trips, stop every two hours to walk around and stretch those legs. If you can't avoid prolonged periods of standing or sitting, rest your veins at least once a day by elevating your legs above your heart.

Avoid wearing tight garments that impede circulation in your legs. No tight stockings (unless they're the specially prescribed elastic stockings that fit your leg precisely), none of those jeans which look like they've been spray painted on, and none of those old fashioned garters that hold up nylons or long socks.

Take good care of your body. Eat well. Put more fiber in your diet. Don't become overweight. Obese people have a huge problem with varicose veins and more serious complications from them. Some doctors won't operate on obese people (typically defined as 20 or more pounds overweight) until they lose weight. Take good care of your feet. It is well known that infections can creep into the bodies of older people (or anyone) because of poor foot hygiene.

Finally, walk more (not in heels but in flat shoes, please, so those calf muscles get a workout.) Climb a few flights of stairs instead of taking the escalator. Jog. Bicycle. Dance. Swim. Do anything but stand or sit still.

■■■■■■■■■■■■■■
GLOSSARY

This glossary of medical terms is offered to help you understand the text of this book and the descriptions of various cardiovascular illnesses of the lower limbs. Some popular terminology is explained within its medical context. However, not all terms defined here are used in this book. They are included because doctors sometimes will use them in explaining a diagnosis or treatment to patients.

abdomen The body cavity located between the chest and pelvis or hip area. From Middle French and Latin.

abnormal Deviating from the normal. From a Latin combination of the prefix *ab-*, "away from," and *normalis*, "normal."

abscess A localized collection of pus. From the Latin *abscedere*, "to go away."

absorb To incorporate within or take up. Originally from the Greek *rhophein*, later the Latin *absorbere*, meaning "to suck up."

acenocoumarol Oral medication whose action delays blood clotting. One of several anticoagulant drugs.

Achilles' tendon The tendon attached to the heel bone and arising from the gastrocnemius and soleus muscles of the calf. Reference comes from Homer's *Iliad,* describing Achilles, whose only vulnerability was in his heel.

acute Rapid or sudden as opposed to "chronic." From the Latin *acutus*, "sharp."

adduct To move a leg or arm, for example, toward the midpoint of the body. From the Latin *adducare*, "to bring together."

adhesion Abnormal connection of different parts of the body to each other; a sinuous band by which parts abnormally adhere to each other; false and unhealthy "connective tissue." From the Latin *adhaerere*, "to stick."

111

adsorption The process by which a substance attracts or takes in another substance; the passage of food in soluble form from the alimentary canal into the bloodstream. From a Latin combination of the prefix *ad-*, "toward," and *sorbeo*, "suck down."

adventitia The external coat of the blood vessel. From the Latin *adventicius*, "coming from the outside."

aeration The exposure of blood to air, such as the process taking place in the lungs. From the Greek *aerios*, "air."

amputation The surgical removal of a limb, or part of a limb. From the Latin *amputare*, "cut around."

anastomosis The joining together of two or more hollow organs. From the Greek *anastomoun*, "to provide with an outlet."

anatomy The study of the structure of the body and the interrelationship of its parts. From the Greek *anatome*, "dissection."

aneurysm Dilation of a portion of the wall of an artery. From the Greek *aneurynein*, "to stretch wide."

angiography X ray of blood vessels after injection of a radio-opaque substance to visually inspect the lumen (interior of a vein or artery) and detect any disease that may be present. From the Greek combination of the prefix *angio-*, "blood vessel," and *graphein*, "to write."

angiology The study of the blood and lymph systems. From a Greek combination of *anggeron*, "vessel," and *logos*, "discourse."

ankle That joint connecting the leg and the foot. From the Old English *ancleow*.

anticoagulant A substance that prevents blood from clotting. A Latin combination of the prefix *anti-*, "against," and *coagulum*, "curdling agent."

aorta The largest artery in the body. It carries blood from the heart to all parts of the body. From the Greek *aeirein*, "to lift."

aperture Opening or orifice to a body cavity or a blood vessel. From the Latin *apertura*, "to open."

apex The top or pointed extremity of a body or organ, such as the apex of the heart. From the Latin word of the same spelling, *apex*, "narrow or pointed end."

aponeurosis A tendon forming a sheetlike membrane. From the Greek *aponeurousthai,* "to pass into a tendon."

areolar Containing minute spaces filled with tissue fluid, areolar connective tissue connects various organ tissues. From the Latin *areola,* "small opening space."

arteriole The small terminal twig of an artery that ends in capillaries. From the Latin *arteriola,* the diminutive of "artery."

artery One of the tubular branching muscular-and-elastic-walled structures that carry blood from the heart to the body. From the Greek *arteria,* "channel."

atrium The upper chambers of the heart. From the Latin word of the same spelling, *atrium,* the central hall of the ancient Roman house.

auricle A portion of the upper chambers of the heart. From the Latin *auricula,* "ear."

autopsy Examination of the human body usually performed to determine the precise cause of death. From the Greek *autoposis,* "act of seeing with one's own eye."

avascular Bloodless, or having very few blood vessels. From a Latin combination of the prefix *a-,* "away from," and *vasculum,* "small vessel."

band In medicine, an adhesion composed of fibrous tissue. From Middle English *bande,* "strip,"

biopsy The removal of tissue for study in order to determine the diagnosis. From the Greek *opsis,* "appearance."

bistoury Slim, surgical knife, frequently used to open an abscess. From the Latin *bis,* "twice," and Middle French *bistorie,* "dagger."

blood platelet Minute blood cells, tinier than the red or white, produced in the bone marrow, that act in clotting of the blood. From the Greek combination *platys,* "broad and flat," and the suffix *-let,* "small."

Buerger's disease Rare, and often confused with "hardening of the arteries," this is a chronic, inflammatory disease of the small arteries of the lower extremities, known medically as "thromboangitis obliterans." This condition can lead to gangrene progressing from the tips of the toes.

bypass   A kind of surgery that involves grafting or attaching a blood vessel or a synthetic tube to an obstructed vein or artery at two points so that blood can flow and pass by the blockage.

calf   The back of the leg below the knee. From the Old English *cealf.*

canal   Any channel or duct of the body, such as the venous channels carrying blood. From the Latin *canalis,* "pipe" or "channel."

canalization   Formation of new channels, for example the reformation of a passageway in a clotted vein following thrombosis of the vessel.

cancer   A malignant, sometimes fatal, tumor, characterized by unlimited, lawless growth, frequently spreading from its site of origin. From the Greek *karkinos,* "crab."

capillary   Minute, thin-walled blood vessels, responsible for feeding the tissues of the body. From the Latin *capillaris,* "hair."

carbon dioxide   Heavy colorless gas in the atmosphere; an end product of metabolism. From a combination of the Latin *carbo,* "coal," the Greek prefix *di-,* "two," and the Greek *oxys,* "sharp."

carcinoma   The medical term for cancer (q.v.). From the Greek *karkinoma,* "cancer."

cardiac   Relating to the heart. From the Greek *kardia,* "heart."

cardiovascular   Relating to the heart and blood vessels.

cartilage   Popularly known as gristle, the elastic, semisoft tissue covering the joints, providing for smooth motion with minimum friction. From the Latin *cartilago,* "wickerwork."

catalyst   Any agent that hastens and stimulates a chemical reaction. From the Greek *katalysis,* meaning dissolution or separation of component parts.

cauterization   Burning by the application of a caustic heat or electric current; the hot iron once used widely in searing wounds to guard against infection or control bleeding. From the Greek *kauterion,* "branding iron."

cavity   A hollow or space within the body or one of its organs. From the Latin *cavus,* "hollow."

cell   The minute protoplasmic masses which make up tissue, such as blood cells, usually each containing a nucleus. From the Latin *cella,* "compartment."

cerebral   Generally referring to the cerebrum, the brain area comprising the higher brain centers. From the Latin *cerebrum,* "brain," believed to have stemmed from the Greek *kara,* "head."

charley horse   Slang for muscle spasm associated with a possible tear of some of the muscle fibers, sometimes with hemorrhage into the substance of the muscle.

chirurgeon   Archaic term for surgeon, still in use in certain formal documents in certain parts of the world. From the Old French *cirurgie,* "surgery."

chronic   Usually of long-term duration, as opposed to acute. From the Greek *chronikos,* "of time."

chronic venous insufficiency   Long-term incompetency of the venous system, characterized by varicose veins leading to one or a series of venous complications.

circulation   The passage of blood from the heart to all parts of the body, plus the return of blood from tissues back to the heart. From the Latin *circulatus,* "circle."

clamp   Surgical instrument used to stop bleeding from severed blood vessels, technically known as a "hemostat." From the Middle Dutch *klampe,* "band" or "fetter."

claudication   Cramplike pain in the leg due to an insufficient arterial blood supply and a symptom of "hardening of the arteries." The pain, usually in the calf, typically occurs after a patient walks, stops when the patient stands still and then strikes again when the patient again walks the same distance (whether that's 200 feet or five blocks). From the Latin *claudus,* "lame," and the verb *claudicare,* "to limp."

clinical   That course of the disease as noted and followed by a physician. From the Greek *klinike,* meaning medical practice at the sickbed.

clot Solidification, or coagulation, of a "ball" of blood within a vein or an artery. From the Old English *clott*.

coagulation The formation of a clot of blood. From the Latin *coagulare*, "to curdle."

collagen A major protein component of skin, tendon, bone, cartilage and connective tissue.

colon That part of the large intestine which connects the small intestine to the rectum.

communicating veins A term often describing the veins that unite the deep and the superficial veins. The term is interchangeable with the perforator veins that connect the saphenous system with the deep system.

congenital Existing from or before birth. From the Latin *congenitus*, "bringing forth."

connective tissue Tissue connecting and holding together cells of an organ; tissues lying between the organs of the body such as the muscles and the blood vessels.

contraceptive A drug or medical device used to prevent pregnancy.

convulsion A violent and involuntary muscle spasm or a series of spasms, sometimes repeated rapidly.

coronary Relating to the heart.

Coumadin An anticoagulant administered as a medication to "thin out" the blood. The generic name is warfarin sodium.

cramp Painful muscular contraction, particularly occurring in the calf muscles at night, often the first symptom of varicose veins. Some researchers think leg cramps at night for pregnant women also can be due to an excess of phosphorus in relation to calcium and suggest cutting back on high phosphorus foods like meat and milk. The word is believed to be traced to the Low German *krampe*, "hook."

cutaneous Generally relating to the outer layer of skin. From the Latin *cutis*, "skin."

cyanosis The bluish or purplish color of the skin, usually the result of insufficient oxygen in the blood. From the Greek *kyanosis*, "dark blue color."

decompensation   Failing circulation of the blood due to faulty heart function, characterized by shortness of breath and irregular heartbeat. From a Latin combination of the prefix *de-* and *compensatus,* "counterbalance."

deep veins   Term that refers to all of the veins beneath the deep fascia connective tissue in the leg.

deep venous thrombosis   The formation of a blood clot, or thrombosis, in the deep veins of the leg.

dermatitis   Inflammation of layers of skin; often a complication of varicose veins, the inflamed skin takes on a red or brownish color. From the Greek *derma,* "skin."

dermatologist   A physician specializing in treatment of skin diseases.

diagnosis   A determination about the nature or cause of a patient's disease or illness. From the Greek *diagignoskein,* "to distinguish."

diaphragm   The muscular membrane separating the chest and abdominal cavity. From the Greek *diaphrassein,* "to barricade."

diastole   The "relaxed" phase of the heart cycle during which the heart chambers fill with blood; the opposite of systole. When blood pressure is measured, the lower number is dystolic pressure. From the Greek *diastellian,* "to expand."

dilated superficial veins   Prominent superficial veins (those closer to the skin) not associated with varicose veins.

disease   An abnormal disturbance in the function of an organ or body structure, such as vascular disease with varicose veins. From the Middle French *desaise,* "trouble."

dissect   To separate tissue. From the Latin *dissecare,* "to cut apart."

diverticulitis   Illness in which sacs on the wall of the large intestine become inflamed.

Doppler   A painless, noninvasive mechanical device used by doctors to measure blood flow in the arteries and veins. Named after a Dutch physicist, it operates by analyzing harmless sound waves that are beamed into the body and bounce back to a microphone. See duplex Doppler analysis.

dorsum   The back of any organ or organ part; also the upper surface, as the dorsum of the foot.

duct   A hollow tube or channel, such as an artery or vein. From the Latin *ducere*, "to lead."

duplex Doppler analysis   A more sophisticated version of the Doppler which sends back pictures in Technicolor (instead of just sound which is recorded on narrow ribbons of paper like ticker tape).

dysfunction   Malfunction or imperfect functioning of an organ or a blood vessel.

eczema   An inflammatory disease of the skin causing itching, redness, sometimes "seeping"; "varicose eczema" usually occurs over a group of long-standing (no pun) varices in the leg. From the Greek *ekzein*, "to erupt."

edema   An accumulation of fluid in the tissues. From the Greek *oidein*, "to swell."

elastic tissue   A type of tissue that is capable of expanding and contracting, found in the lining layers of the veins and arteries.

embolism   The obstruction of a vein or an artery by a blood clot usually broken off from a larger clot in some part of the circulatory system. From the Greek *emballein*, "to insert."

embolus   The blood clot, or thrombus, becomes an embolus as it breaks off and migrates through the bloodstream.

endothelium   Membranous cells which form the inner lining of blood vessels, lymph channels and various cavities of the body. From the Latin *endothelia*, "layer."

epidemiology   The scientific study of the occurrence and prevalence of diseases, particularly those associated with contagion. From the Greek *epidemia*, "visit" or "epidemic."

ERT   Estrogen Replacement Therapy. Formerly recommended for menopausal women to relieve hot flashes, vaginal dryness and other discomforts associated with the tapering off of menstrual cycles. Replaced by HRT or Hormone Replacement Therapy, which involves the use of progesterone as well as estrogen.

estrogen   The female sex hormone manufactured by the ovaries. From the Greek *oistros,* "frenzy."

etiology   The study of the cause of disease.

evolution   The process by which higher, more complex life has developed from more primitive and simpler forms.

excision   To cut out or off surgically; removal of veins, for example. From the Latin *excidere,* "to cut."

expiration   Exhalation or breathing out. From the Latin *espirare,* "to breath out."

extensor muscles   Those muscle that straighten out a limb or a part; flexor muscles bend or flex a limb or a part of the limb.

extravasation   The act of body fluid leaving its normal channels and flowing into the surrounding tissues. From a Latin combination of the prefix *extra-,* "outside," and *vasculum,* "small vessel."

fallopian tubes   Canal on either side of the uterus; passageway through which the egg or ovum is carried from the ovary to the uterus. Names for Gabriel Fallopius (1523–1562), Italian anatomist credited with its discovery.

familial varicose veins   Sometimes called primary varicose veins, they are the most common type and often connected with hereditary or family tendencies. Affecting (1) the greater saphenous system, (2) the short saphenous system. From the Latin *familia,* "family."

fascia   Connective tissue found throughout the body, wrapping or enclosing muscles, nerves and blood vessels. From the Latin *fascia,* "bundle."

femoral vein   A major vein in the upper thigh that gets blood from the saphenous vein and feeds it to the iliac vein in the pelvis.

femur   Popularly known as the thighbone; the large bone connecting the hipbone to the knee bone. From the Latin *femur,* "thigh."

fertilization   The union of an egg and a sperm cell in sexual reproduction. From the Latin *ferre,* "to carry" or "to bear."

fetus   Referring to the unborn child in the later stages of pregnancy; during the first three months of pregnancy, the fetus is known as the embryo.

fever   Elevation of body temperature above the normal 98.6 degrees Fahrenheit or 37 degrees Celsius.

fibrin   A protein substance that forms a kind of net in the body. The net traps blood cells near injured tissue and helps to form a clot that stops the bleeding.

fibrinogen   Protein manufactured in the liver; forms fibrin during the clotting process.

fibula   The thinner of two leg bones extending from the outside of the knee to the outer side of the ankle. From the Latin *fibula,* "clasp."

fissure   A narrow slit or cleft on or in a part of the body; break in the skin. From the Latin *fissum,* "cleft."

fistula   An abnormal canal or pipelike opening in some part of the body, often leading to an internal organ. From the Latin *fistula,* "pipe."

flexor muscle   In general, muscle that bends a limb. Any muscle that flexes a joint. From the Latin *flexus,* "bend."

follicle   Small gland from which secretions arise; for example, the graffian follicles which secrete an egg from an ovary. From the Latin *follis,* "bag."

foot   The terminal part of the leg. From the Old English *fot.*

fossa   Shallow pit or depression in the contour of an organ, bone or other part of the body. From the Latin *fossa,* "pit" or "depression."

gangrene   Literally, death of tissue, most often the result of an insufficient blood supply to the area. From the Greek *gangraina,* "gnawing."

gastrocnemius muscle   The main calf muscle in the back of the lower leg which is responsible for extending the foot and flexing the leg. From a Greek combination of the prefix *gastro-,* "belly" and *nemius,* "two heads."

gauze   Material used in the dressing of surgical wounds or to sponge and "dry" wounds following surgery. From the Middle French *gaze,* "thin material."

gene   That part of a special germ cell which determines inherited characteristics such as blood type and hair color. There are thousands of genes transmitted on each of the 23 pairs of chromosomes that everyone has in each cell in the body.

genus   A type, class or group in the description of living objects marked by one or more common characteristics. From the Latin *genus*, "birth."

germ   Bacterium or microorganism capable of or with the potential of producing disease. From the Latin *gignere*, "to beget."

gonad   A sex gland. The reproductive sex glands in women are the ovaries; in men, they are the testicles. From the Greek *gonos*, "sex gland."

gout   Painful disease characterized by joint inflammation, caused by faulty metabolism; arthritis-related condition distinguished by excess uric acid in the body. From the Middle English *gutta*, "drop."

graft   Skin or tissue taken from one part of the body to replace defective tissue in another; vein or artery grafts performed to "skip over" a vascular occlusion involve attaching or grafting a vessel above and below the obstruction.

groin   The area between the front of the thigh and the abdomen. From the Old English *grynde*, "abyss."

hamstring muscle   Powerful muscle in the back of the thigh that bends the knee.

heart   The hollow muscular organ in the chest which by its rhythmic contraction acts as a pump maintaining the circulation of the blood throughout the body. From the Old High German *herza*.

hematologist   A specialist in diseases of the blood and blood forming organs. From the Greek prefix *haemo-*, "blood."

hematoma   Hemorrhage with the formation of a blood clot.

hemorrhage   Escape of blood from a blood vessel. From the Greek *haimorrhagia*, "severe discharge of blood."

hemorrhoids   Varicose veins of the rectum or anus mucous membrane. From the Greek *haimostasis*, "styptic."

heparin   A drug that prevents blood from clotting. From the Greek *hepar,* "liver."

heredity   Transmission of qualities from ancestor to descendant; the passage of bodily characteristics or disease from parent to offspring. From the Latin *hereditas,* "heir."

Hg   Chemical symbol for mercury.

hip   Region on either side of the pelvis; joint where the upper end of the thighbone and the pelvic bones meet. From the Greek *kybos.*

history   In medicine, the recording of the patient's symptoms relating to the sequence of events pertaining to an illness. From the Latin *historia,* "knowing," taken from the Greek *eidenai.*

hormone   A chemical produced by a gland, secreted into the bloodstream and affecting cells or organs elsewhere in the body. From the Greek *horman,* "to stir up."

HRT   Hormone Replacement Therapy. A mix of estrogen and progesterone, usually recommended for menopausal women seeking relief from the discomforts of menopause or perimenopause (the period leading up to menopause).

humor   Any normal fluid within the body; in early medicine, the factor governing health and disease. From the Latin *humere,* "to be moist."

hygiene   Science that deals with health and its preservation; observation and practice of health standards. From the Greek *hygies,* "healthy."

hyper-   Prefix meaning "excessive" or "above"; e.g. hypertension, which is tension or pressure above normal. From the Greek *hyper,* "over."

hypo-   Prefix meaning "too little." From the Greek *hypo,* "under" or "below."

hypodermic   Instrument for use in injections beneath the skin. From the Latin *hypoderm,* "under the skin."

ibuprofen   Generic name for a pain killing drug that treats inflamed tissues.

iliac vein A major vein in the pelvis that connects the leg veins to the inferior vena cava.

iliofemoral Pertaining to the ilium and the femur, i.e., as in that area or joint where the leg bone joins the hip bone.

ilium The broad upper part of the hipbone. From the Latin *ilia*, "hip area."

incipient Earliest beginnings.

indigenous Native to an area.

induration Quality of being hard; abnormally hard tissues. From the Latin *induratio*, "hard."

inferior vena cava The venous trunk for the lower extremities and for the pelvic and abdominal viscera. It begins at the level of the fifth lumbar vertebra by union of the common iliac veins, passes upward on the right of the aorta, and empties into the right atrium of the heart.

inflammation A condition characterized by redness, pain, heat and swelling. From the Latin *inflammare*, "to set on fire."

infusion The injection of a solution, generally into a vein. From the Latin *infundere*, "to pour into."

inguinal region The lower part of the abdominal wall. From the Latin *inguinalis*, "groin."

injection The act of introducing a medication or other substance into the body. From the Latin *injectus*, "to throw into."

inoperable A condition that precludes surgery. From a Latin combination of the prefix *in-*, "not" and *operatus*, "performing."

intercellular tissue Tissue situated between cells.

interstitial Pertaining to, or situated within. From the Latin *interstitus*, "standing still in the middle."

intima The innermost lining of an artery or a vein. From the Latin *intimus*, "well inside."

intramural Situated within the walls. From a Latin combination of *intra-*, "within" and *murus*, "wall."

ischemia   Inadequate blood supply to an organ or an extremity. From the Greek *echein,* "to hold."

ischium   The bone on which one's weight is borne in the act of sitting. The dorsal and posterior of the three principal bones composing either half of the pelvis. From the Greek *ischion,* "hip joint."

lactic acid   A hydrogen-carbon-oxygen compound manufactured in the body as an end product of sugar metabolism. From the Latin *lactus,* "milk," and *acidus,* "pointed" or "strong."

lancet   Small, pointed, two-edged surgical knife, its extra-sharp point used primarily for puncturing. From the Latin *lancea,* "knife."

latent   Not immediately obvious; concealed. From the Latin *latens,* "hidden."

lateral   To the side, as opposed to toward the midline. From the Latin *lateris,* "side."

lesser circulation   The pulmonary circulation, flow of blood from the heart to the lungs and from the lungs back to the heart; as opposed to the systemic circulation, which carries the blood to all parts of the body.

lethal   Deadly or final, as a lethal or terminal disease. From the Latin *letum,* "death."

leukocytes   The white blood cells with characteristic cell nuclei; a colorless amoeboid (one-celled) mass, as a white blood corpuscle. From a Greek combination of *leukot,* "white," and *kytos,* "cell."

ligaments   Tough connective tissue holding bones together; strong band of tissue connecting bones or supporting large interior organs. From the Latin *ligare,* "to tie" or "to bind."

ligation   Tying off of blood vessels during the performance of surgery; the application of a ligature. From the Latin *legatus,* "a tying up."

ligature   Material used for tying off a blood vessel.

loin   The flank or area just below the ribs to the side of the body; the part of the back between the thorax and the pelvis. From the Latin *lumbus,* "loin."

lumbar region   The lower part of the back. From the Latin *lumbus,* "loin."

lumen   The passageway inside a hollow organ, such as the lumen of a vein or an artery. From the Latin *lumen,* "light" or "air shaft."

lymph   The fluid traveling through the lymph channels. From the Latin *lympha,* "water," derived from the Greek *nymphe,* "nymph."

lymphedema   Abnormal swelling of a limb caused by the blockage of the lymph channels. The lymph system is comparable to the vascular system minus the heart, artery and vein components. From a Latin combination of *lympha,* "water," and *oidema,* "swelling."

malignant   Virulent, tending to go from bad to worse, even to lethal. From the Latin *malignitas,* "ill will" or "malice."

malleolus   The rounded bony projection of the ankle; laterally, the bony knob protruding from the outer ankle, the medial malleolus is the protuberance on the inner side of the ankle. From the Latin *malleus,* "little hammer."

marrow   Tissue inside the bone. From the Old English *mearg* and Old High German *marag,* "marrow."

massage   Usually the rubbing and kneading performed to relax tired, aching or painful leg muscles; medically, systematic therapeutic friction. From the French *masser,* "to massage," derived from the Arabic *massa,* "to stroke."

media   The middle tunic or coat of an artery, a vein or a lymph vessel. From the Latin *medius,* "middle."

melanin   The brown pigmentation of the skin. From the Greek *melas,* "black."

melanocyte   A pigment cell containing melanin.

membrane   A thin layer of tissue that covers or ensheaths a surface or divides an organ. From the Latin *membrana,* "skin" or "parchment."

menopause   Popularly called the change of life. Known technically as the climacteric, the time of a woman's life when her menstrual period stops. From a combination of the Greek prefix *meno-,* "month," and the French *pause,* "hesitation."

menstruation   In a woman, the discharge, approximately once a month except during pregnancy or menopause, of a bloodlike fluid from the uterus. From the Latin *menstruus,* "monthly."

metabolism   The process by which food components are broken down and transformed into elements that are utilized by the body for energy and/or growth. From the Greek *metaballein,* "to change."

metatarsus   The long bones of the foot. From a Greek combination of the prefix *meta-,* "among," and *tarsus,* "flat of foot."

milk leg   Popular and ancient name for the swollen leg condition that often follows an attack of phlebitis, frequently associated with pregnancy; medically phlegmasiaalba dolens.

mm   Millimeter.

myositis   Inflammation of muscle.

necrosis   Death of tissue, usually due to faulty nutrition to that tissue area. From the Greek *nekroun,* "to make dead."

nervus   Commonly, a mole on the skin. Discolored patch on the skin due to pigmentation. From the Latin *naevus,* "mole on the skin."

nitrates   Group of chemicals that cause dilation of blood vessels and the lowering of blood pressure. From the Greek *nitrin,* derived from the Egyptian *ntry,* "element."

nucleus   The central portion of the cell. From the Latin *nucleus,* "kernel."

obesity   Overweight, excessive accumulation of fat in the body. From the Latin *obedere,* "to eat up."

obliterate   In medicine, to close off, like an occluded vein. From the Latin *oblitterare,* "to efface."

occlusion   Shutting off, as blood flow within a clotted vein.

operable   A condition indicating that a patient can benefit by surgery; the opposite of inoperable.

oral   Referring to medication taken by mouth, such as an orally administered anticoagulant or birth control pills. From the Latin *ora,* "mouth."

organ A body part performing a specific function. From the Greek *organon,* "a tool" or "an instrument."

osteomyelitis Infection of the bone. From the Greek *osteon,* "bone."

osteoporosis The loss of bone density that affects some women during and after menopause.

ostium Opening, entrance to an organ or bodily structure. From the Latin *ostium,* "door."

ovarian follicle A sac or cavity within an ovary containing an egg; every month these follicles burst to release the egg. From the Latin *ovum,* "egg."

ovulation The process during which an egg is released from an ovary.

ovum Female reproductive cell; the Latin word for egg.

parietal Of or pertaining to the walls of a cavity, as the parietal peritoneum, which lines the abdominal cavity. From the Latin *paries,* "wall."

patella The kneecap. From the Latin *patina,* "shallow dish."

patent Wide open, such as the lumen of a blood vessel. From the Latin *patere,* "to open."

pathology Science dealing with the study of diseases. From the Greek *pathologia,* "the study of emotions."

perforating veins Also known as perforators or communicating veins. Veins that perforate or pass through the deep fascia to connect the superficial veins with the deep veins. Often referred to as communicating veins because they allow the two venous systems to keep in touch. Valves within these veins control the direction of blood flow.

perimenopause Early stages of menopause.

periosteum The tissue forming a sheath around the bone. From the Greek *periosteon,* "around a bone."

peripheral The surface, outward part. From the Greek *peripherein,* "to carry around."

peritoneum   The thin lining of the abdominal or peritoneal cavity. From the Greek *peritonanion*, "stretched around."

peroneal region   The region roughly on the outer side of the lower leg. From the Greek *perone*, "fibula."

phagocyte   Microscopic cells with the capability of fighting harmful bacteria or other body invaders. From the Greek *phagein*, "to eat," and *kytos*, "cell."

phlebectomy   The surgical excision or removal of a vein. From a Greek combination of the prefix *phleb-*, "fluid," and *extos*, "out."

phlebitis   An inflammation of a vein lining.

phlebogram   See **venogram**.

phlebothrombosis   The presence of a blood clot or thrombus in a vein. From the Greek *thrombos*, "clot."

pigmentation   The deposit of coloring matter in the skin; a frequent complication of varicosities, particularly around the ankle area. From the Latin *pingere*, "to paint."

plasma   The fluid component of circulating blood, minus the red and white blood cells. From the Greek *plaussein*, "to mold."

platelet   Thrombocyte; tiny colorless disk in the circulating blood, an important factor in blood clotting. From the Greek *platys*, "broad or flat."

polidocanal   An anesthetic widely used in Europe in sclerotherapy.

popiteal vein   A major vein behind the knee that drains blood from the calf area and directs it to the femoral vein in the thigh. It is part of the deep system of veins in the legs.

posterior   Situated in the back, or toward the rear of an organ or other part of the body. From the Latin *posterus*, "after."

post-operative   A period of time following surgical procedures.

pouch   Any anatomical region that forms a pocket or sac. From the Middle English *pouche*, "sac."

Premarin   A pharmaceutical medication that contains estrogen, a female hormone.

progesterone   A female hormone created by the ovaries to prepare the uterus to receive a fertilized egg.

progestin   A crude form of progesterone and the term used for progesterone-like substances that are made synthetically.

progestogen   A synthetic substance that acts somewhat like progesterone in the body.

prophylaxis   In medicine, measures carried out to help ensure health or prevent disease. From the Greek *prophylaktikos,* "keeping guard up."

prosthesis   An artificially replaced body part. From the Greek *prostithenai,* "to add to."

protein   A substance in certain foods that contains nitrogen, a nutrient found in all animal and vegetable tissue. From the Greek *protos,* "first."

pulmonary circulation   Referring to the flow of blood to and from the heart via the lungs.

pulse   The wave of movement felt when a finger is pressed over an artery. The beat or wave is caused by heart contractions. Normally, every heartbeat will create a pulse beat. From the Latin *pulsus,* "beat."

recanalization   The natural reopening of a blood vessel, blocked by a blood clot, as following phlebitis. From a Latin combination of the prefix *re-,* "back" or "again," and *canalis,* "little pipe."

regimen   A planned treatment for an illness or disease such as a daily treatment or orders prescribed by the doctor to alleviate the discomfort of varicosities. From a Latin *regare,* "to rule."

respiration   The act of breathing. From the Latin *respirare,* "to inhale and exhale."

retrograde   Moving in the opposite direction of normal, as "retrograde flow" of blood falling back in a vein, usually the result of incompetent valves. From the Latin *retrogradus,* "going back."

revascularization   The reestablishment of efficient flow of blood to an organ or a limb. From a Latin combination of the prefix *re-,* "back" or "again," and *vasculum,* "small vessel."

sacrum Shield-shaped bone composed of five fused vertebrae situated at the base of the vertebral column, forming the back wall of the pelvis. From the Latin *os sacrum*, "last bone of spine."

saphenous veins Veins in the leg that drain blood from the superficial leg veins. The greater saphenous is the longest vein in the body; it runs from the foot to the groin. The lesser saphenous goes from the outside of the foot to popiteal vein behind the knee.

scalpel Surgical cutting instrument, a straight blade with a convex cutting edge. From the Latin *scalpellum*, "small chisel" or "knife."

sclerosis Deposit of fibrous tissue replacing the original softer structure to produce a hardening deposit such as sclerosis of the arterial walls. From the Greek *skeroun*, "to harden."

sclerotherapy Injection of medication into a vein to cause clotting in order to obliterate the lumen, such as in the injection treatment of varicose veins. From a Greek combination of *skeroun*, "to harden," and *therapeutikos*, "treatment."

sepsis A toxic condition resulting from infection. From the Greek *sepsis*, "decay."

sequelae Development in the course of a treatment or therapy; progression of a disease; the complication of varicosities. From the Latin *sequela*, "following."

serum The portion of blood persisting after coagulation. From the Latin *serum*, "whey."

sheath Tissue covering of the blood vessels or veins. From the Old High German *sceida*.

shock Condition of the body caused by an inadequate amount of blood circulating due to hemorrhage. From the Middle Dutch *schocken*, "to jolt."

shunt An abnormal union between blood vessels; in surgical procedure, an operation in which the blood is detoured so it can bypass occluded blood vessels. From the Middle English *shunten*, "to flinch."

sign Physical evidence of disease or the potential for a diseased state. Various "signs" in medicine can pinpoint a problem. "Homan's

Sign," for example, can reveal thrombosis of the deep veins of the legs. From the Latin *signum,* "mark" or "sign."

sinus   Any abnormal hollow cavity in the body, generally connecting to the outside. From the Latin *sinus,* "curve" or "hollow."

Sotradecol   A drug used by doctors in sclerotherapy.

spasm   An abrupt and forceful contraction of a muscle, sometimes lasting several minutes or longer and characterized by severe pain. From the Greek *spasmos,* "drawing" or "pulling."

sphincter   Ring-like muscle that controls the opening and closing of a body passage, such as controlling blood flow into and away from a vein or artery. From the Greek *sphinkter,* "band."

spider bursts   Small red-blue venules in the skin of the legs and feet that can be a serious complication of varicose veins. From the Greek *histasthai,* "to stand."

striated   Primarily describing human muscle, striated or striped muscle that controls voluntary movement. From the Latin *stria,* "funnel," "channel," or "groove."

stripping   Surgical procedure for the correction of varicose veins in which the vein is removed by a "stripper," a metal instrument inserted into the lumen of the vein to be removed. From the Middle English *strippen,* "to remove."

subcutaneous   Beneath the skin, as the subcutaneous veins, or the saphenous systems. From the Latin *subcutaneus,* "hidden beneath the skin."

superficial   As opposed to deep. From the Latin *suficies,* "lacking in depth" or "pertaining to the surface."

superficial veins   All the veins situated in the subcutaneous fatty layer of tissues, such as the great and lesser saphenous system of veins.

superior   Anatomically, situated in a higher region of an organ or part of the body. From the Latin *superus,* "upper."

suppurate   To form exuding pus, as an infected and irritated ulcer might develop. From the Latin *suppurare,* "to form pus."

symptom A sign or evidence of an ailing or diseased condition in a patient. A patient diagnosed as "symptomatic" has all the common symptoms of a disease. From the Greek *symptoma*, "a happening."

syndrome A group of signs or symptoms recognized as forming a definite pattern of a specific condition or a disease in a patient. From the Greek *syndrome*, "a combination."

systemic Applying to (1) a condition or disease involving the entire body of a patient or (2) the general circulatory system of blood flow throughout the body as apart from the pulmonary or "lung centered" system.

systole The contraction phase of the heart which expels blood, forcing it onward through the body.

tarsus The instep of the foot including its seven bones; the portion of the human foot between the metatarsus and the leg. From the Greek *tarsos*, "wickerwork."

telangiectasis Reddish areas appearing on the skin of the leg that are caused by stretching and dilation of venules and arterioles.

tendon The rough band of dense whitish fibrous tissue that connects a muscle with another organ of the body, such as bone, responsible for the force that the muscle exerts. From the Latin *tendere*, "to stretch."

therapy Relating to treatment of an illness, disease or disorder. From the Greek *therapeuein*, "to treat."

thrombectomy The surgical removal of a blood clot obstructing a vein or artery. From the Greek *thrombos*, "clot."

thrombin An enzyme that aids in the clotting of blood by converting fibrinogen to fibrin.

thromboangiitis obliterans Known more simply as Buerger's disease, it is an inflammation of the arteries or veins, and if left untreated, it can result in gangrene of a finger or toe. From a combination of the Greek prefix *thrombo-*, "clot," the Greek suffix *-angio*, "blood vessel," and the Latin *oblitterare*, "to be in the way of."

thrombocyte Technical word for blood platelets, that component critical in the normal blood clotting process.

thrombophlebitis An inflammation of the vein lining that includes the presence of a clot.

thrombosis The formation of a blood clot in a vein or an artery; the ailment of the abnormal blood clotting and obstruction. From the Greek *thrombos,* "clot."

thrombus A clot of blood formed within a blood vessel.

tibia Larger of two major leg bones, situated in the inner side of the leg. From the Latin *tibias,* "tibia" (between the knee and the ankle).

tissue A collection or aggregation of cells that are similar in type. From the Latin *textere,* "rich, woven fabric."

tonicity The state of relaxation or contraction of a muscle; the property of possessing "tone" or healthy vigor of the muscles and the body. From the Greek *tonikos,* "tension" or "tone."

tortuous Containing many turns and twists, such as an enlarged varicose vein. From the Latin *torquere,* "to twist."

tourniquet Instrument or procedure for controlling abnormal bleeding or hemorrhage. From the Old French *torner,* "to turn."

toxin Poisonous substance manufactured within the body by harmful bacteria; able to initiate antibody or antitoxin formation within the body. From the Greek *toxikon,* "arrow poison."

transplant Living tissue usually taken from one part of the body (or blood vessel) and affixed to another; at times, a graft. From the Latin *transpantare,* "to plant across or over."

triangle A triangular shaped area of the body, such as the femoral or the inguinal triangle. From the Latin *triangulum,* "three sided."

ulcer A crater other than a wound on the surface of the skin or on the interior lining of a hollow organ; the base of the crater is often inflamed and red. From the Greek *helkos,* "wound."

ulcer, varicose One specifically associated with, and usually a complication of, a worsening varicose vein condition.

unilateral Pertaining to one side of the body; "bilateral" refers to both sides of the body or to affecting both limbs or organs, such as bilateral involvement of the legs. From a Latin combination of the prefix *unus-*, "one," and *laterialis*, "side."

Unna boot A semisolid, paste-like and gaiter-shaped covering that is made up of healing components and applied to the lower leg and upper part of the foot to encourage healing of ulcers. (The heels and toes are uncovered.) The device was developed at the end of the nineteenth century by the German dermatologist Paul Gerson Unna (1850–1929) in Hamburg.

uric acid Normally, a chemical compound of the blood; it is elevated in a metabolic disease called gout. From the Greek *urina*, "urine."

uterus Anatomical term for the womb, the hollow organ that is a home for the fetus for nine months before birth. From the Latin *uterus*, "belly."

vacuolar Applying to a vacuole, a clear space within a cell. From the Latin *vacuus*, "empty."

valsalva maneuver A technique doctors use to look for malfunctioning vein valves in the lower extremities. Patients are asked to hold their breath and bear down, tensing the abdominal muscles and thereby increasing venous blood pressure throughout the lower extremities.

valve A device that controls the flow of liquid. Vein valves in the legs force blood to work against gravity and by directing its flow up the body back to the heart.

varicose As applied to veins, those that are stretched, dilated and tortuous appearing. Source experts offer various etymological origins. Most agree it is adapted as used from the Latin *varicosus*, "full of dilated veins"; some feel the affixed Greek suffix *-osis*, "condition," points to a Greek origin. (Traces also have been made to the Lithuanian word *viras*, "measles of swine.") Finally, others believe it is derived from the old Arabic word for vine.

varicosities Veins that are dilated and tortuous, including "stretched" superficial veins.

varix Term for varicose veins, generally singular. From the Latin *varix*, "swollen vein."

vascularization The formation of new blood vessels.

vascular system The system of blood vessels including the arteries, veins and capillaries.

vasodilatation The dilation of a vein or an artery.

veins Those blood vessels that carry blood from the tissues back to the heart for purification. From the Latin *vena*, "deep water channel."

vena cava The two largest veins in the body are the inferior vena cava, which carries blood from the lower extremities, and the superior vena cava, which carries blood from the upper extremities into the heart.

vena comitans A vein accompanying its corresponding artery.

venogram An X ray of a vein, taken following the injection of an opaque substance into the vein to outline its course. A diagnostic procedure used to determine the presence of varicose veins or a block within a vein.

venous stasis Abnormal slowing of blood flow within a vein. From the Latin *vena*, "deep water channel," plus *statis*, "standing" or "stopping."

ventricle Chamber of the heart, from which blood is rhythmically forced into the arteries. From the Latin *ventriculus*, "belly."

venules Small veins that connect capillaries to larger veins. These are effectively the feeder roads that direct deoxygenated blood to the main highway veins en route back to the heart.

warfarin An anticoagulant crystalline compound administered to ward off blood clotting in patients who have suffered thrombosis.

white leg See **milk leg.**

X rays Electromagnetic rays of short wave length with the power to penetrate body tissues. Also called Roentgen rays, named for their discoverer, Wilhelm Conrad Roentgen (1845–1923), distinguished German physicist.

■■■■■■■■■■■■■■■■■■■■■■■■■■■■■■
SUGGESTED READINGS

Following are the names of books that are worth consulting. The list of books is followed by some articles that are noteworthy but not specifically mentioned at the end of any chapter.

Allen, Edgar, Nelson Barker, and Edgar Himes. *Peripheral Vascular Diseases*. Philadelphia and London: W. B. Saunders Co., 1962.

Behrman, S.J., and Robert W. Kitsner (editors). *Progress in Infertility*. Boston: Little Brown & Co., 1968.

Bergan, John J., and James S.T. Yao. *Venous Problems*. Chicago: Year Book Medical Publishers, Inc., 1978.

Berger, Andrew J. *Elementary Human Anatomy*. New York, London, Sydney: John Wiley & Sons, Inc., 1967.

Brooks, Stewart M. *The Sea Inside Us*. New York: Meredith Press, 1968.

Burkitt, Denis P. and H.S. Trowell (editors). *Refined Carbohydrate Foods and Disease*. London, New York, San Francisco: Academic Press, 1975.

Camp, John. *Magic, Myth and Medicine*. New York: Taplinger Publishing Co., 1974.

Cleave, T.L. *On the Causation of Varicose Veins*. Bristol, United Kingdom: John Wright & Sons, Ltd., 1960.

Coney, Sandra. *The Menopause Industry: How the Medical Establishment Exploits Women*. Alameda, Ca.: Hunter House, 1994.

Dodd, Harold, and Frank B. Cockett (editors). *The Pathology and Surgery of the Lower Limb*. Edinburgh, London: Churchill, Livingstone, New York. 1976.

Fegan, George. *Varicose Veins/Compression Therapy*. London: William Heineman Medical Books, Ltd., 1967.

Goldman, Mitchel P. *Sclerotherapy Treatment of Varicose and Telangiectatic Leg Veins*. St. Louis, Missouri: Mosby Year Book, Inc., 1991.

Green, David. *Queen Anne*. New York: Charles Scribner's Sons, 1970.

Hackett, Francis. *The Personal History of Henry the Eighth*. New York: Norden Library, 1929.

Hatcher, Robert. *Contraceptive Technology*. New York: Irvington Publishers, 1994.

Lacey, Robert. *The Life and Times of Henry VIII*. London: Praeger Publishers, 1972.

Majno, Guido. *The Healing Hand/Man and Wound in the Ancient World*. Cambridge: Harvard University Press, 1975.

Morrell, Roger M. *Thrombophebitis*. New York, London: Grune & Stratton, 1963.

Nachtigall, Lila, and Joan Rattner Heilman. *Estrogen: The Facts Can Change Your Life*. Los Angeles: The Body Press, 1986.

Reitz, Rosetta. *Menopause: A Positive Approach*. New York: Penguin Books, 1977.

Scarisbrick, J.J. *Henry VIII*. Berkeley, Los Angeles: University of California Press, 1968.

Seeman, Bernard. *The River of Life*. New York: W. W. Norton & Company, Inc., 1961.

Thorwald, Jurgen. *The Century of the Surgeon*. New York: Pantheon Books, 1957.

Thorwald, Jurgen. *Science and Secrets of Early Medicine*. New York: Harcourt, Brace and World, Inc., 1963.

White, Paul Dudley. *My Life and Medicine*. Boston: Gambit, Inc., 1971.

Articles

"Dietary Supplements" in *Consumer Magazine*, published by the U.S. Food and Drug Administration, Washington, D.C., November 1993.

Kost, Kathryn, Jacqueline Darroch Forrest, and Susan Harlap. "Comparing the Health Risks and Benefits of Contraceptive Choices." *Family Planning Perspectives*, March/April 1991.

"The Menopause, Hormone Therapy and Women's Health," published by The Office of Technology Assessment, U.S. Congress.

Mosher, William. "Contraceptive Practices in the United States, 1982–1988" *Family Planning Perspectives*, Sept./Oct. 1990. (This magazine is published by the Alan Guttmacher Institute in New York, which makes reprints available.)

"Taking Vitamins: Can They Prevent Disease?" in *Consumer Reports*, September 1994.

Index